Racism in Psychology

Racism in Psychology examines the history of racism in psychological theory, practice and institutions.

The book offers critical reviews by scholars and practising therapists from the US, Africa, Asia, Aoteoroa New Zealand, Australia and Europe on racism on the couch and in the wider socio-historical context. The authors present a mixed experience of the success of efforts to counter racism in theory, institutions and organisations and differing views on the possibility of institutional change. Chapters discuss the experience of therapists, anti-Semitism, inter-sectionality and how psychological praxis is part of a colonialist project.

The book will appeal to practising psychologists and counsellors, socially minded psychotherapists, social workers, sociologists and students of psychology, social studies and race relations.

Craig Newnes is editor of the *Journal of Critical Psychology, Counselling and Psychotherapy* and has published numerous book chapters and academic articles. He has been Chair of the BPS Psychotherapy Section and was director of one of the UK's largest NHS psychological therapies departments. He has also edited and authored over a dozen books. He has spoken at numerous events as a critic of psychology and has given seminars at many UK and international universities.

Racism in Psychology

Challenging Theory, Practice and Institutions

Edited by Craig Newnes

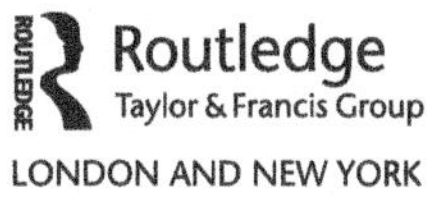
Routledge
Taylor & Francis Group
LONDON AND NEW YORK

First published 2021
by Routledge
2 Park Square, Milton Park, Abingdon, Oxon OX14 4RN

and by Routledge
605 Third Avenue, New York, NY 10158

Routledge is an imprint of the Taylor & Francis Group, an informa business

British Library Cataloguing-in-Publication Data
A catalogue record for this book is available from the British Library

Library of Congress Cataloging-in-Publication Data
Names: Newnes, Craig, editor.
Title: Racism in psychology: challenging theory,
practice and institutions / edited by Craig Newnes.
Description: 1 Edition. | New York: Routledge, 2021. |
Includes bibliographical references and index. |
Identifiers: LCCN 2020051572 (print) | LCCN 2020051573 (ebook) |
ISBN 978-0-367-63503-9 (hardback) | ISBN 978-0-367-63502-2 (paperback) |
ISBN 978-1-003-11940-1 (ebook)
Subjects: LCSH: Racism–Psychological aspects. |
Race relations–Psychological aspects.
Classification: LCC BF175.4.R34 R335 2021 (print) |
LCC BF175.4.R34 (ebook) | DDC 155.8/4–dc23
LC record available at https://lccn.loc.gov/2020051572
LC ebook record available at https://lccn.loc.gov/2020051573

ISBN: 978-0-367-63503-9 (hbk)
ISBN: 978-0-367-63502-2 (pbk)
ISBN: 978-1-003-11940-1 (ebk)

Typeset in Bembo
by Newgen Publishing UK

Printed in the United Kingdom
by Henry Ling Limited

With gratitude and love to my family and other teachers – you know who you are and only a few of you know how much learning you offer.

Contents

List of contributors ix
Foreword by Nimisha Patel xii

PART I
Institutional racism 1

1 Race, racism and the psy project 3
CRAIG NEWNES

2 Invisible anti-semitism in psychology 16
KATE MIRIAM LOEWENTHAL

3 The global system of white supremacy within UK clinical psychology: an African psychology perspective 26
ERICA MAPULE MCINNIS

4 Re-embedding racism in psychology: indigenising the curriculum in Australian psychology 43
PAUL DUCKETT

5 'Something less terrible than the truth': *Oliver Twist* and anti-semitism 57
JONATHAN CALDER

6 Racism and the rights movement 69
LAUREN TENNEY

PART II
Race, theory and practice 85

7 Racism and learning disabilities 87
DEBORAH CHINN

8 Judaism and the psy project 100
CRAIG NEWNES

9 Racism in New Zealand psychology, or, would Western psychology be a good thing? 110
PIKIHUIA POMARE, JULIA IOANE, AND KEITH TUDOR

10 Counselling the 'other' 131
CEMIL EGELI

11 I refuse to choose: culture, trans-culturalism and therapy 147
SIM ROY-CHOWDHURY

12 Echo to authenticity: exploring identity in an age of privilege and supremacy 160
DWIGHT TURNER

13 Embracing the kaleidoscope: talking about race and racism in clinical psychology 176
STEPHANIE HICKS AND CATHERINE BUTLER

Name index 192
Subject index 194

Contributors

Catherine Butler is a clinical psychologist and systemic psychotherapist currently working at the University of Bath as clinical director and deputy head of department.

Jonathan Calder lives in Leicestershire and has written for *The Guardian* and *New Statesman*. He blogs at Liberal England.

Deborah Chinn is a clinical psychologist with the King's College London and Wandsworth Community Learning Disability Healthcare Team.

Paul Duckett is a critical community psychologist who is presently working in an academic role at CQUniversity Townsville, Australia. His research and teaching has focused on disability issues in general and health issues in particular and this has involved him working with users of psychological services and governmental organisations to promote the rights of disabled people. He collaborates with other critical scholars to examine and lay bare the cultural and political factors that impact psychologised understandings of so-called mental health and disability, mainstream theories and practices of psychology and reconstructed histories of psychology.

Cemil Egeli is a senior lecturer and programme leader for counselling skills (BA combined hons) at the University of Chester. He is studying for a PhD at Warwick University using autoethnographic and biographical methods to explore the mixed cultural experiences of students in Health Education. He also works as a counsellor and previously worked as a secondary school music teacher.

Julia Ioane is a first-generation New Zealand-born Samoan. She is a clinical psychologist and senior lecturer in the clinical psychology programme at Massey University, Auckland, Aotearoa New Zealand.

Stephanie Hicks is a newly qualified clinical psychologist working in Community CAMHS in South Oxfordshire.

Kate Miriam Loewenthal is Emeritus Professor of Psychology at Royal Holloway, London University and is currently a Visiting Professor at Glyndwr University, Wales, and New York University in London. Her research has focused on mental health in minority groups in the UK. She is interested in how religious factors relate to mental health, and is currently working both on spirituality in trauma therapy, and on anti-semitism. She has been involved in providing and evaluating culture-sensitive mental health support services. She has published several books including *Religion, Culture and Mental Health*, 2007, and co-edits the journal *Mental Health, Religion and Culture.*

Erica Mapule McInnis is a Chartered Clinical Psychologist (UK) and Founder, Director and Principal Clinical Psychologist for Nubia Wellness and Healing (www.nubiawellnessandhealing.co.uk). She developed the first African Psychology Emotional Wellness School online in the UK, is a Churchill Fellow (2016) and was awarded post-fellowship funding to develop 'Know Thy Self – Adinkra Cards' (an African-centred therapy engagement tool with diverse applications). She has 22 years NHS (National Health Service) experience and is an occasional lecturer for university clinical psychology training programmes. Recent speaking engagements on African Psychology include Kensington Royal Palace (London), The High Commission for Trinidad and Tobago (Belgravia, London), a Mental Health Foundation (MHF) Podcast (aired July 2020) and BBC Radio 4 (award-winning 'Black Girls Don't Cry', 2019). She is a professional member of the Association of Black Psychologists (ABPsi) and is Black British of Jamaican parentage.

Craig Newnes is a Consulting Critical Psychologist and Compassionate Conversationalist, ex-Director of Psychological Therapies for Shropshire's Mental Health (NHS) Trust, dad, grandad, editor, author and co-director of Egalitarian Publishing. He is an ex-chair of the British Psychological Society Psychotherapy Section and edited *Clinical Psychology Forum* for 19 years. He has published numerous book chapters and academic articles and is Editor of the *Journal of Critical Psychology, Counselling and Psychotherapy.* His books include *Clinical psychology: A critical examination* from PCCS Books and the edited volumes: *Making and breaking children's lives; Spirituality and psychotherapy; This is madness: A critical look at psychiatry and the future of mental health services; This is madness too: A further critical look at mental health services.* His latest books are *A critical A to Z of electroshock* (2018), *Children in society: Politics, policies and interventions* (2015), *Inscription, diagnosis, deception and the mental health industry: How psy governs us all* (2016), the co-edited *Teaching critical psychology* (2018) as well as *52 ways to survive a pandemic* and *52 ways to change your life* (both 2020)

Pikihuia Pomare is a clinical psychologist, lecturer and affiliate of the Centre for Indigenous Psychologies in the School of Psychology, Massey University, Aotearoa New Zealand.

Sim Roy-Chowdhury is a clinical psychologist and systemic psychotherapist and until recently has been a Clinical Director at East London Foundation Trust. He is involved in the clinical psychology doctoral programmes at the University of East London and the University of Hertfordshire. His PhD research analysed family therapy sessions using discourse analysis. He is interested in the creation of versions of psychology and psychotherapy practice that are located within the social, cultural and political contexts within which people live their lives.

Lauren Tenney, PhD, is a psychiatric survivor and activist based in New York. She was first involuntarily committed at age 15. Her work aims to expose the institutional corruption which is a source of profit for organised psychiatry, and to abolish state-sponsored human rights violations, such as murder, torture and slavery (www.laurentenney.us).

Keith Tudor is professor of psychotherapy at Auckland University of Technology, Aotearoa New Zealand. He is also a Teaching and Supervising Transactional Analyst.

Dwight Turner is Senior Lecturer within the School of Applied Social Sciences at the University of Brighton, lecturing on their PG Dip and MSc courses in Counselling and Psychotherapy, a PhD Supervisor at their Doctoral College, a psychotherapist and supervisor in private practice, and a part-time lecturer at the Centre for Counselling and Psychotherapy Education (CCPE) in London. He completed his PhD through the University of Northampton and the CCPE in 2017. His phenomenological and heuristic study used transpersonal and creative techniques such as visualisations, drawing and sand play work to explore the unconscious intersectional nature of privilege and otherness. An activist, writer and public speaker on issues of race, difference and intersectionality in counselling and psychotherapy, Dr Turner can be contacted via his website (www.dwightturnercounselling.co.uk).

Foreword

Nimisha Patel

As a trainee clinical psychologist – in the 1980s – two questions in particular plagued me and I grappled with them, soon realising that this Sisyphean task could only lead to despair. The first question was where is race and racism in psychology? Indeed, this seemed a rhetorical question since racism was everywhere and palpable to those attuned to it and versed in defending against its toxic forces. The second question was why was racism not mentioned, but instead the construct of culture employed, attributed to the other, serving to deflect attention from the normative gaze, whilst at the same time silently, powerfully entrenching and justifying racism.

In exploring racism within psychology, and tracing its historical and current manifestations, the contributors in this book tackle those questions in varying ways, starting with a stark analysis of the racist and colonising history of psychology, or more specifically, the employment of psychology as part of enduring colonisation projects of countries such as the UK. The manifestations of the global system of white supremacy (McInnis, Chapter 3) in UK clinical psychology are perhaps a more apt description for institutional racism, and in taking an African psychology viewpoint, McInnis offers an exciting vision of what psychology could be, 40 years hence, 'if the past was different' (p. 26). The past is not different, however, and very much present, 'alive and kicking' in our theories, models, training, practices, research, therapies, and in our psychological services. Amongst a range of perspectives on different forms of racism, and racisms, authors offer their insights into 'what if …' – what if we could imagine a different psychology, what if we could adopt African models of psychology and enrich and transform psychological practices, what if we could move beyond essentialist notions of culture and race and see and work with complexity better, what if our curriculum could be reformed, etc.

The book brings hope, whilst simultaneously dashing those hopes, punctuating 'aha' moments for the reader with 'yes, but …' Indeed, my own journey in clinical psychology, as a trainer, researcher, clinician, service manager, etc., and my own experiences of racism, direct and indirect, subtle and not so subtle, have taught me that optimism needs more than unbridled hope and a desire to do things differently. As some authors highlight – undoing racism is more than decolonising the curriculum, interrogating history and our own values and worldviews; it requires courage to ask why and how do we find ourselves where we are (still not that different to 30 years ago); it requires us to ask what did we each do, or not do, to keep us where we are; and to ask, can we face the racist history of psychology, can we reimagine it, and are we the right or only people who can do this? Duckett's argument (Chapter 4) that a formal apology by the Australian Psychological Society to Indigenous Australians, which included an acknowledgement of the ways in which psychology had been complicit in the marginalisation of Indigenous peoples in Australia, is necessary, but the de-politicisation and lack of recognition of the need for political change amounts to much of the same – a paternalistic embedding of a racist agenda in the psychology curriculum. In psychology, then, change requires us to move beyond acknowledgement and an apology, or a tinkering with psychology's racist history – it demands a radical overhaul of psychology. The question is, are we up for this? My hope is yes, but optimism tempered with the enduring bitter taste of institutional racism reminds me to try, yes, but with all of us together, our eyes wide open: this is a long-haul and bumpy journey which will outlast the present generation of psychologists, psychology students and trainees, but we must keep trying; the past is no excuse for more of the same in the future.

Part I

Institutional racism

Chapter 1

Race, racism and the psy project

Craig Newnes

Summary

This chapter examines some of the racist and colonialising history of psychology. It highlights the ways in which psy practitioners are professionaliaed into narrow forms of theory and praxis that can neglect culture, religion and diversity. The outcome is an impoverishment of experience for practitioners and a lack of relevance for service recipients.

Cross-cultural studies of so-called depression by researchers in the industrialised regions presuppose a dichotomy of mind and body and related theory of emotion. Emotions are, however, not constituted the same way in different cultures; the anthropologist Clifford Geertz, for example, regarded ideas *and* emotions as cultural artefacts (Geertz, 1973).

Anthropologists and cross-cultural psychologists argue that affects are inseparable from cultural systems of meaning. It has been suggested that culturally informed models of what might be described as depression should investigate indigenous or ethno-psychological models of dysphoric affects. Themes include factors such as indigenous categories of emotion, the predominance of particular emotions within societies and ethno-physiological accounts of bodily experience of emotions (Jenkins et al., 1991). Conceptions of emotion are embedded within notions of self, characterised as varying along a continuum between egocentric and socio-centric. Individuals with a more socio-centric sense of self are considered to be more relationally identified with others than those with a more egocentric sense of self, who try to function as individuals. The former have often been associated with non-Western/indigenous cultural traditions, the latter with traditions attuned to post-industrial materialism.

An understanding of emotions as intrapsychic events, feelings or introspections of the individual (rather than the individual, community or ancestors) is predominantly a Western conceptualisation. The Ifaluk of Micronesia don't conceptualise thoughts and emotions solely within the individual. Rather, these can be found in relationships between persons or within events and situations. The Pintupi peoples of Australia have a kin-based conception of self in contrast to people following more westernised traditions where self is seen as constituted by individuality. For example, in White, middle-class, affluent, communities it tends to be individual children who are marked as depressed rather than families or communities, although there is an increasing acknowledgement amongst psychology practitioners that poor housing, persistent assaults on one's character and sense of self due to a system of institutional racism, decrepit infrastructure and poverty create environments where the experience of *opp*ression is frequently identified as *de*pression, albeit depression identified as individual distress.

Whether attempting to heal individuals or communities some 80% of the world's population includes herbs, dance, incantation and prayers to ancestors or gods and different forms of spirituality. Since 3000 BCE Ayurvedic medicine has emphasised the importance of three doshas: Vata, Pitta and Kapha (tripartite systems are also integral to Western notions underlying, for example, psycho-analysis and cognitive behaviour therapy; see Chapter 8, this volume). In Ayurveda, disease and illness originate from an imbalance in the three energies and a disconnection from nature (again, the notion of imbalance can be found in Western traditions from humoral theory to the metaphor of 'brain biochemical imbalance'). Amongst other ills Ayurveda is used for: Alzheimer's disease, fear and being overwhelmed, asthma, cancer, dementia and high blood pressure.

African psychology uses the best of African culture, thinking, practices and rituals in constant exchange with the world for betterment (Karenga, 2010). The philosophies of the Nile Valley and ancient Egypt feature prominently (Browder, 1992; Nobles, 2006) in addition to an abundance of diverse African cultural principles with contemporary derivatives (Parham, 2002). These raise spiritual, emotional and physical resonances for dispersed intergenerationally oppressed people, potentially enabling self-understanding, endurance, betterment, progression and transformation (Akbar, 2017; Akbar, 1998; Nobles, 2006; Parham, 2002). Becoming inspired by traditional African culture during therapy conversations can include reflecting on proverbs or sayings familiar to particular families or communities, which represent strategies for dealing with life situations and traditional wisdom. This can include the use of Ananse stories (Ananse is a folktale character taking the form of a spider with the spirit of wisdom and all knowledge of stories) and traditional West African wisdom concepts such as Adinkra symbols as tools for wellness (Adom et al., 2016) (see Chapter 3, this volume).

The 7,000-year-old history of Judaism involves prayer and the role of rabbi/*rebbe* who counsels after the *gabai* (rebbe's assistant) has met with people and then: 'After interviewing the supplicant about his family, his background and his troubles, the gabai delivers the *kvitl* [written description of the presenting problem] and an oral report to the rebbe' (Zborowski & Herzog, 1995, 172). This might be seen as analogous to a psychiatric intake session or psychological assessment carried out in the first session (see Chapter 8, this volume).

These early paragraphs cannot do justice to the wealth of understanding and healing represented within cultures different from the overwhelmingly white hegemony to be found in theories and practice underlying much of modernist psy in Northern industrial global regions. The consequences for people not fitting the arbitrary norms of a psychology dominated by individualism and capitalism have been considerable.

Psychology and racism

Between 1900 and 1939 British eugenicists included the psychologists Burt, Spearman and Pearson (holder of the inaugural Galton chair in eugenics at University College, London). Writing on Beyondism, the eugenics movement he founded, the US psychologist Cattell (progenitor of Cattell's 16 PF Personality Inventory) claimed:

> The vast majority of humans on the planet are 'obsolete' and … the earth will be choked with the more primitive forerunners unless a way is found to eliminate them … Clarity of discussion … would be greatly aided if genocide were reserved for a literal killing off of all living members of a people … and genthanasia for what has been above called 'phasing out,' in which a moribund culture is ended, by educational and birth control measures.
>
> (Cattell, quoted in Mahler 1997)

Cattell was writing just over 60 years ago, some 27 years *after* the Holocaust. Intellectuals such as the socialist Webbs, Havelock Ellis and George Bernard Shaw as well as the black shirts of Oswald Moseley were all eugenicist.

Notions of unbounded 'spectrum disorders' and 'family histories' of madness can be positioned alongside the eugenic thrust of the first half of the last century. 'Risk' of inheritance of certain so-called disorders is now a standard assumption in psychiatry and underlies UK protocols for tests and scans of potentially Down's Syndrome foetuses carried out in ante-natal clinics. In combination with the idea of a disorder spectrum and the desirability of 'health' (for the purposes here defined as a comfortable life and the absence of debilitating illness) screening foetuses is equivalent to screening children and, where deemed necessary, inscribing then prescribing to those children (Newnes, 2016).

Although Terman developed the Terman-Merrill Index (an early measure of IQ) as a means of offering specific schooling to 'less educable' children, he was less sanguine in his approach to race: 'Dullness seems to be racial – psychologists and their IQ tests are the beacon light of the eugenics movement.' (Terman, 1930).

Tasked with selecting suitable military entrants, the psychologist Brigham had this to say, 'Our data indicate clearly the intellectual superiority of the Nordic race group' (Brigham, 1923). Fears of 'degeneration' of the gene pool led, in the US, to forced sterilisation of thousands of – frequently poorly educated – African Americans who scored poorly on the Binet-Simon tests of intelligence. As recently as the 1970s, black people were argued to be intellectually inferior to white people by scientists in the USA such as William Shockley (Shockley 1971).[1]

Colonizing psychology

In 1858, Forbes Winslow, editor of the *Journal of Psychological Medicine*, protested that asylums and their inmates could be 'brought into the market and offered for sale, like a flock of sheep, to the highest bidder' (Winslow, quoted in Parry-Jones, 1972, 88). Changes in asylum management in Britain in the nineteenth century (a 'takeover' of public and private institutions by qualified medical personnel) were matched in India. The subcontinent had seen a form of institutional psychiatry based on the profit motive. Run by the East India Company, asylums catered for European woman, soldiers and sailors, as well as the Indian and Eurasian insane. The latter were kept in conditions described as 'abominable'. The officials insisted on separation by race, class and gender, leading to considerably better living conditions for Europeans. By the turn of the century, an assistant surgeon, Valentine Connolly, ran a private madhouse in Madras while W. Dick owned Bengal's private asylum (for Europeans). By the 1840s the Madras asylum was structurally unsound and Connolly made a fortune from its sale (and, *de facto*, the sale of its inmates). In the Calcutta asylum the quality of provision was entirely based on social standing and racial background. For over 50 years the purchase and sale of asylums (and their inmates) in India made handsome profits for those in similar positions to Connolly.

Despite the conditions within the company's asylums, 'cure rates' bear comparison with those claimed in England at the time. The lowest rate claimed, for example, for Calcutta in the 1840s was 12%, while English and Welsh military and naval asylums were claiming 11%. Mortality was a different matter: by 1850 the mortality for the Bengal asylum had reached 18% whereas in England the rate was half that (Ernst, 1991). Conspicuous by its absence was any acknowledgement or use of Indian healing practices predating by millennia the European method. Europeans were the elite so, by definition, indigenous medicine was inferior.

Founded in 1916, the first Indian psychology department opened in Calcutta University and the Indian Psychological Association was formed in 1925. Indian academic psychology was influenced by early British Psychological Society praxis and structure. According to Clay (2002), 'Convinced of the universal applicability of Western psychology, many Indian psychologists tried to keep the discipline free of any Indian traditions.'

'India Education', a website promoting careers in the humanities positions psychology in an exclusively westernised way, with no acknowledgement of the diversity of spiritual and cultural customs within a population exceeding a billion people. The following paragraph would be familiar to any UK clinical psychologists training in the 1960s:

> Psychology is the study of human behavior and mental processes. Psychologists study a person's reactions, emotions, and behavior, and apply their understanding of that behavior to treat the associated

> behavioral problems. Treatment is focused on therapy and counselling … Psychologists are therefore responsible for identifying psychological, emotional, and/or behavioral issues, as well as diagnosing any specific disorders, by using information gleaned from patient interviews, patient's tests and records, and medical reference materials. Clinical psychologists … may act as therapists for people who are experiencing normal psychological crises (e.g., grief) or for individuals suffering from chronic psychiatric disorders.
> (www.indiaeducation.net/careercenter/humanities/psychology/)

Barnette's summary of his observations following a tour of Indian clinics and universities in the early 1950s included a view that clinicians were 'preoccupied with the Rorschach, and TAT [Thematic Apperception Test]', a phenomenon that would have been familiar to observers in the US and UK in the second half of the twentieth century (Barnette, 1955, 120). It appears that the next half century brought little change; when Professor of Psychology Mark Rapley visited Hyderabad a decade ago he was taken aback (possibly to the UK in the 1960s) to find that clinical psychologists on psychiatric wards were wearing white coats.

Referring to Barnette's findings, Misra and Rizvi (2012) suggested the establishment of a national licensing board of psychology to conduct written and oral examinations for credentialing clinicians, the license to be renewed every two years contingent upon up to 25 hours of continuing education (post-masters level degree) including three to four hours' training in professional ethics. In the absence of a subcontinent-specific diagnostic nosology the authors recommend, 'diagnosing mental disorders using the current edition of a standard diagnostic system, like, DSM-IV-TR (American Psychiatric Association, 2000), or ICD-10 (World Health Organization, 1993)'. Rather than assuming validity for culture-specific concepts of distress, the authors suggest, 'a need for a verifiable and replicable body of data demonstrating not only incremental validity of using Indian concepts but also, inapplicability of Western concepts in India'. Consistent with the Western popularity of 'evidence-based' therapies the authors suggest that practitioners 'consider' using CBT, DBT or M-CBT. They add, 'clinical psychology in India appears to have flirted with a "soft" romantic view of mental disorders. There is need to strengthen the empirical base for diagnosing and treating mental illness within a comprehensive framework of professional ethics and code of conduct.' (Misra & Rizvi, 2012). Misra is based in private practise in Ohio.

The Indian Association of Clinical Psychology (IACP) was formed in 1968 with a view to advancing concepts of mental health and the profession of clinical psychology (see www.iacp.org.in). Published twice annually since 1974 the Association's *Indian Journal of Clinical Psychology* mostly eschews both culturally informed articles or more recent developments in UK clinical psychology, such as the Reflective Practitioner, Psychological Formulation or Power Threat Meaning frameworks. The first of the two 2019 issues includes unapologetically diagnosis-based articles on behaviour modification, ADHD, schizophrenia, mild mental retardation, alcoholism and Social Anxiety Disorder. A wide-ranging editorial on suicide, covering social factors, sociological and psycho-analytical analyses, neurotransmitter theories and more, does refer to religious and cultural strictures. It opens, 'Suicide is the most heinous crime committed by the victim himself' (Sengar, 2019).

An internet forum (http://IndianPsychologists@yahoogroups.co.in) was started in November 2006 (Manickam, 2008). There are over 4,000 members. Commenting on the website Misra and Rizvi note, 'one is nostalgically reminded of informal groups of people in coffee-houses, wayside tea-stalls, and village-well or river-banks providing a non-judgmental platform to exchange thoughts and opinions' (Misra & Rizvi, 2012, 23).

Funded by the Chinese Association of Science and Technology the Chinese Psychological Society was founded in 1921 and now has over 9,000 members. The aim of the society is to 'unite psychologists throughout the country, to develop academic activities, and to promote research and exchange, in order to accelerate the development of psychological science, so as to contribute to China's social development'. The society publishes two journals, *Acta Psychologica Sinica* and *Psychological Science* (http://resources.iupsys.net/iupsys/index.php/iupsysresources/133-china-articles/3838-chinese-psychological-society).

The CPS has 15 professional committees covering specialties that include Industrial Psychology, Medical Psychology, Military Psychology, Personality Psychology, Psychological Measurement and Counseling Psychology. The *first* Ethic Codes for Psychological Assessment were issued in 1993 – over 70 years after the society's formation.

In October 2011, representatives from the society met with American Psychological Association (APA) staff; the two organisations signed a Memorandum of Understanding 'to facilitate future exchange and interaction' (*APA Monitor*, 2012).

Like their Indian counterparts Chinese psychologists cannot be accused of a lack of ambition; a grouping with less than 10,000 members aspires to influence in a country of one and a half billion souls. Claiming a scientific agenda the CPS hopes to influence a country dominated by folk religion or Taoism. Estimates of religious adherence in China vary and are difficult to verify due to factors such as the essentially familial basis of religion and corresponding lack of organisational structures in addition to the official suppression of religious practice during the cultural revolution. Estimates thus vary from 11 to 30% of the population as practicing Buddhists while some 23.8% are said to worship gods and ancestors. A conservative estimate might be that half the population – perhaps 750 million people – follows forms of folk religion more keenly than they might ascribe to modernist forms of psy science.[2]

Adair compares the process of indigenization in India and Taiwan highlighting the role of language. For Adair, the language of science is a technicalised form of English; the language of culture may be Hindi, Mandarin, Spanish or

German. He notes a psychologist interviewed in India about indigenization of psychology who says, 'As a psychologist I think in English; but as a person I feel in Hindi.' He suggests that indigenous research is likely to be 'more successful' if it is conceptualised and the data are collected in the native language (Adair, 2004).

And ...

In terms of qualified UK clinical psychologists a letter in *The Psychologist* notes that, 'research by the Health & Social Care Information Centre in 2013 showed that Black, Asian and Minority Ethnic (BAME) individuals make up only 9.6 per cent of qualified clinical psychologists in England and Wales, in contrast to 13 per cent of the population' (York, 2020).

The discipline has accepted mostly white applicants for training despite attracting many culturally diverse applicants. One survey a decade ago found the acceptance rate for (overwhelmingly white) women to be 85 per cent of applicants (Turpin & Coleman, 2010). The profession, unlike medicine and veterinary science, has consistently failed to change its ethnic profile. Strategies to increase diversity have been put forward since at least 1989 (see Davenhill et al., 1989, and Bender & Richardson, 1990). Since 1998, courses have made some alterations to selection criteria in an attempt to increase diversity while developing teaching materials to 'raise awareness' of cultural diversity (Patel et al., 2000).

In 1991 the UK's Division of Clinical Psychology (DCP) formed a Special Interest Group in Race and Culture Issues as part of this process. It eventually was titled the Special Interest Group in 'Race' and Culture and became a Faculty.

A comparison may be made with the state of the profession in the US. Graduate programmes in psychology were originally closed to women and members of ethnic minority groups. Between 1879 and 1920 10,000 doctorates were awarded in psychology; 11 of these went to Black students. In the following half-century (to 1966), of 3,767 doctorates awarded, eight went to African Americans (Albee, 1969). Subsequent to the formation of the Association of Black Psychologists (ABPsi) in 1968 and associations for Hispanic, American Indian and Asian American psychologists, the American Psychological Association created a Board of Ethnic Minority Affairs in 1980. By 1986 there was a Division-Society for the Psychological Study of Ethnic Minority Issues. Numbers of Black and minority ethnic psychologists increased. The impact of the Historically Black Colleges and Universities (HBCU) (which in times of segregation accepted and trained black students) should not be underestimated. The HBCU not only provided institutions primed for later generations of Black students to attend, but often had Black lecturers and courses set up to meet their needs.

In 1986 there were 16,519 clinical psychologists with PhDs in the US; 505 were Hispanics, American Indians and African-Americans (a total of 3%). For the African Americans involved (159), this was a 20-fold increase over the previous 60 years (Heckler, 1986). Three years later the proportion of Black and minority ethnic students being awarded PhDs in clinical psychology had risen to 10% of the total. This may reflect changes in access for education amongst Black and minority communities, policy changes on the part of the APA (Mays & Albee, 1992) and the work of associations such as ABPsi.

In the UK, DCP-sponsored strategies to increase the proportion of trainees from Black and ethnic minority backgrounds have borne little fruit. Following the initial report in 1989 cited above there were regular surveys and projects (see, for example, Bender & Richardson, 1990; British Psychological Society, 2004; Turpin & Fensom, 2004). Ten years ago Turpin and Coleman (2010) concluded that in relation to psychology and diversity, 'the road to hell was paved with good intentions'. A British Psychological Society (BPS) 'action plan' was drawn up but not monitored. A further BPS Professional Practice Board action plan was not implemented. In fact it was superseded by the Equalities Policy of the BPS. There was also a 'diffusion of responsibility' (Turpin & Coleman, 2010) across three DCP subgroups (the Group of Trainers, the Special Interest Group in Race and Culture and the Managers' Faculty). *Clinical Psychology and Diversity: Progress and Continuing Challenges* reveals that in the ten years 1994–2004 the average acceptance rate for applicants to training from 'non-white' backgrounds was 6.2%. The last four years of the time period reviewed saw an average acceptance rate of 8%. Between 2004 and 2009 this figure increased to 9.6%, a rise the authors describe as 'extremely disappointing' (Turpin & Coleman, 2010).

Based on an analysis of Clearing House Data applications for clinical psychology training places, those identifying as white British are twice as likely to be accepted as those from Black and minority ethnic backgrounds and three times as likely as those identifying as Black (Murphy, 2019).

It is tempting to analyse the lack of substantive change in the area of diversity in terms of the usual suspects: institutionalised racism, a changing political and governmental context which leaves all but the most administratively well-resourced professions unable to respond quickly enough to policy change at national level, the amount of BPS work taken on by a relatively small number of members who mostly have full-time (academic) employment and the slowness of large bureaucracies enmeshed in other large bureaucracies. It is equally possible to suggest that the goal of achieving a supposedly 'more representative workforce' is misguided; the historical Euro-centricity of clinical psychology theory and praxis (a concern repeatedly raised by groups such as the DCP Special Interest Group in Race and Culture) creates too great a challenge if attempting to make such praxis 'fit' a more diverse population. Perhaps, as Mays and Albee have commented when discussing psychotherapy, clinical psychology is something for white middle-class professionals to be delivered by white middle-class professionals. Mays and Albee note that ethnic minorities, whatever their character, community and creative strengths are more likely to be poor, live in substandard housing, suffer educational disadvantages and other examples of discrimination. At the same time they are more likely to suffer a wide range of physical health problems, from increased tooth decay to cirrhosis. Citing, amongst others, Flaskerud, they suggest that members of ethnic minorities more often seek help from traditional healers, root doctors, clergy, herbalists and family and friends. By contrast there are more psychotherapists per capita in Washington, DC, than anywhere else in the world – the majority from the white area of Northwest Washington (Mays & Albee, 1992).

Whether or not the reader concurs with Mays and Albee's rather dour proposal for limiting psychotherapy to the white middle classes, the lack of change in UK clinical psychology since 1989 would suggest that the profession has been unable to achieve its stated goals, though *reiterating* those goals is now part of professional praxis. The profession is faced with a paradox. Wedded to a philosophy of individualism, yet expecting that theories, research and psychological therapies can be generalised, it might conclude, *pace* Sartre, that 'Hell is other people' because everyone is different. It is a position the profession resists.

An approach growing alongside mainstream clinical psychology's lack of change is the establishment of organisations attempting to offer culture appropriate forms of help and healing to non-White groups. The Black, African and Asian Therapy Network (BAATN), for example, claims to be the UK's largest independent organisation, 'specialising in working psychologically, informed by an understanding of intersectionality, with people who identify as Black, African, South Asian and Caribbean'. The Network aims 'To ensure people of Black, African, South Asian, Caribbean and People of Colour have the resources available to them through which they can psychologically liberate themselves and live their lives more fully according to their ideals' (BAATN www.baatn.org.uk/).

It cannot be assumed that any culture is monolithic. Just as there are several different forms of Hinduism and Judaism, identifying as white, Black or Asian does not give the observer access to what the person means by these terms. The person may or may not know something of the cultural history behind whatever identifier she uses. White UK psychologists may know that the courts of England from the eleventh to the fourteenth centuries spoke French and laws were written in French and Latin. Equally, they may not and might view the history of England as a kind of seamless progression from Roman rule to the modern day. Learning something of history is invariably enlightening – knowing something of other cultures and their disparate histories equally so. One irony of the lack of a committed approach on the part of clinical psychology and its training community to BAME diversity is that little is learnt of BAME, Judaic, Hindu and other forms of healing. Instead, clinical psychology sinks under the weight of modernist scientism, a culture grounded in culturally specific dinosaurs like cognitive behaviour therapy and diagnosis and a preoccupation with 'the individual'.

But ...

The search for multi-culturalism in psychology is hardly new. Pittu Laungani (1936–2007), for example, caused something of a stir in the field of cross-cultural counselling and psychotherapy. He saw client-centred counselling (a reflective Western approach) as unsuited to those from India, who would favour a more directive approach to therapy, with guidance and advice (a position reflected in the Indian Psychological Society's statement of purpose; see Newnes, 2018). For Pittu, the Western approach to psychotherapy tended to operate on a horizontal model and assumed equality, whereas an Indian model would be vertical, with the therapist as the guru or guide.

He suggested an East/West counselling bridge resting on eight pillars or dimensions, four Western and four Eastern – individualism and communalism; cognition and emotionality; free will and determinism; materialism and spiritualism.

A recent special issue of *Clinical Psychology Forum* (2019) places racism under the gaze, as do articles by McInnis (2017), Ackah (2020) and Bellesi et al. (2020). To know about the racist roots of psychology, both in its institutions and praxis, may, however, be a purely academic exercise when studying or working in contexts that privilege white, heterosexist theories and practice. Undergraduate psychology teaching remains wedded to individualism and theories of internality rather than community. Post-graduate clinical psychology teaching may well emphasise context or human rights (see, for example, the Liverpool and University of East London programmes) but a question remains whether thousands of years of cultural meaning should become an add-on to modernist psy or *replace* it. Clinical psychologists offering services to people with different cultural and ethnic backgrounds to themselves are almost *forced* to rely on theories and methods incompatible with the position of the other. For practitioners from, for example, an observant Jewish background, leaving work before sunset on a Friday in winter may be easily accommodated. Would that same practitioner have been exposed to the Jewish roots of Western psychological theory and practice (see Chapter 8, this volume) in their training? Do trainee clinical psychologists get exposed to African origins of psychology (see, for example, James, 1954/2013; Hilliard, 1995) in a useful and informed manner? Do lecturers bring a cross-cultural critique to bear when presenting material on, say, Dialectical Behaviour Therapy or the inscription of autism? Again, as an academic exercise, these ideas are not so difficult.

Judy Ryle (2020) suggests that the first step for the discipline is apology. In the case of UK psy that apology could mirror that of the Australian Psychological Society made to Aboriginal and Torres Strait Islander people, acknowledging psychology's role in contributing to the erosion of culture and to their mistreatment (Carey et al., 2017).

Acknowledging white privilege would require more than a critique of and apology for psychology's racist past and contemporary role in oppression.

A structural change (at least in the UK) might involve changes to the current committee structures of the DCP. This has the advantage of being in the control of the discipline, although the process would, no doubt, be beset by contextual obstacles. For example, there are no BAME, White or religious faculties. Instead the faculties focus on identified (or inscribed) populations – Older People, Eating Disorders, Addictions and so on. These divisions reflect arbitrary service groupings rather than acknowledging (and celebrating) inter-sectionality.

In pursuing a more culture sensitive path, however, clinical psychology runs the risk of being overtaken by a potentially lethal degree of soul-searching and, as an individualistic endeavour, bound to fail.

Acknowledgement

My thanks to Erica McInnis for comments and contributions.

Notes

1 In 1978 my friend Audrey Campbell, a woman with no less than three doctorates and immense personal authority, finally had enough of living in New Orleans when told by a white woman to sit at the back of a Greyhound bus.

2 http://en.wikipedia.org/wiki/Religion_in_China#Statistics Accessed: 31 August 2020.

References

Ackah, W. (2020). There are fewer than 100 black professors in Britain – why? *Clinical Psychology Forum, 325*, 13–14.

Adair, J. J. (2004). Creating indigenous psychologies: Insights from empirical social studies of the science of psychology. In K. Uichol, Y. Kuo-Shu, & H. Kwang-Kuo (Eds.). *Indigenous and cultural psychology: Understanding people in context.* New York: Springer Science Business Media, pp. 467–485.

Adom, D,, Asante, E. A., & Kquofi, S, (2016). Adinkra: An epitome of Asante philosophy and history. *Research on Humanities and Social Sciences*, vol. *6*(14), 42–53.

Akbar, N. (1998). *Know Thy Self.* Tallahassee, FL: Mind Productions.

Akbar, N. (2017). *New Visions for Black Men.* Tallahassee, FL: Mind Productions,

Albee, G. W. (1969). A conference on the recruitment of Black and ethnic minority students and faculty. *American Psychologist, 24,* 720–723. https://doi.org/10.1037/h0027864

APA Monitor (2012) APA and Chinese Psychological Society: Furthering interaction and exchange *APA Monitor, 43,* 1, 13.

Barnette, W. L. (1955). Survey of research with psychological tests in India. *Psychological Bulletin, 52,* 105–121.

Bellesi, G., Sarfraz, J., Manley, J., Tekes, S., Basit, H., & McNulty, N. (2012). Why do Black Carribean women benefit less from talking therapies? A pilot study in an inner London IAPT service. *Clinical Psychology Forum, 326,* 24–29.

Bender, M., & Richardson, A. (1990). The ethnic composition of clinical psychology in Britain. *The Psychologist, 2*, 250–252.

Black, African and Asian Therapy Network. www.baatn.org.uk/ Accessed 28 August 2020.

Brigham, C. (1923). *A Study of American Intelligence*. Princeton, NJ: Princeton University Press.

British Psychological Society. (2004). *English Survey of Applied Psychologists in Health and Social Care in the Probation and Prison Service*. Leicester: British Psychological Society.

Browder, A. T. (1992). *Nile Valley Contributions to Civilization: Exploding the Myths*, vol 1. Hyattsville, MD: Institute of Karmic Guidance.

Carey, T. A., Dudgeon, P., Hammond, S. W., Hirvonen, T., Kyios, M., Roufeil, L., & Smith, P. (2017). The Australian Psychological Society's apology to Aboriginal and Torres Strait islander people. *Australian Psychologist, 52, 4*, 261–267 https://doi.org/10.1111/ap.12300 see also: www.psychology.org.au/About-Us/who-we-are/reconciliation-and-the-APS/APS-apology.

Clay, R. (2002) An indigenized psychology. Psychologists in India blend Indian traditions and Western psychology. *American Psychological Association Monitor*, May, *33*, 5.

Clinical Psychology Forum. (2019). Special issue: Racism. *CPF, 323*.

Davenhill, R., Hunt, H., Pillary, H. M., Harris, A., & Klein, Y. (1989). Training and selection issues in clinical psychology for black and minority ethnic groups from an equal opportunities perspective. *Clinical Psychology Forum, 21*, 34–36.

Ernst, W. (1991). *Mad Tales from the Raj: The European Insane in India 1800–1858*. London: Routledge.

Flaskerud, J. H. (1986). The effects of culture-compatible intervention on the utilization of mental health services by minority clients. *Community Mental Health Journal, 22*(2), 127–141. https://doi.org/10.1007/BF00754551.

Geertz, C. (1973). *The Interpretation of Cultures*. New York: Basic Books.

Heckler, M. M. (1986). *Report of the Secretary's Task Force on Black and Minority Health. US Department of Health and Human Services.* Washington, DC: US Government Printing Office.

Hilliard, A. G. (1995). *The maroon within us. Selected essays on African American community socialization*. Baltimore, MD: Black Classic Press.

India Education. www.indiaeducation.net/careercenter/humanities/psychology/ Accessed 31 August 2020.

James, G. G. M. (1954/ 2013). *Stolen legacy*. New York: Start Publishing.

Jenkins, J., Kleinman, A., & Good, B. (1991). Cross-cultural studies of depression. In J. Becker & A. Kleinman (Eds.). *Psychosocial Aspects of Depression*. 1st ed. (pp. 67–100). Englewood Cliffs, NJ: Lawrence Erlbaum Associates Inc.

Karenga, M. (2010). *Introduction to Black Studies*. 4th ed. Los Angeles, CA: University of Sankore Press.

Manickam, L. S. S. (2008). Research on Indian concepts of psychology: Major challenges and perspectives for future action. In K. R. Rao, A. C. Paranjpe, & A. K. Dalal (Eds.), *Handbook of Indian psychology* (pp. 492–505). Cambridge: Cambridge University Press.

Mays, V. M., & Albee, G. W. (1992). Psychotherapy and ethnic minorities. In D. K. Freedheim (Ed.). *History of psychotherapy: A century of change* (pp. 552–570). Washington, DC: American Psychological Association.

McInnis, E. M. (2017). Black psychology: A paradigm for a less oppressive clinical psychology. *Clinical Psychology Forum, 299,* 3–8.

McInnis, E. M., & Moukam, R. R. (2013). Black psychology for Britain today? *Journal of Black Psychology, 39*(3), 311–315. doi:10.1177/0095798413480663.

Mehler, B. (1997). Beyondism: Raymond B. Cattell and the new eugenics. *Genetica, 99, 2–3,* 153–163. 29. doi: 10.1007/BF02259519

Misra, R. K., & Rizvi, A. H. (2012) Clinical psychology in India: A meta-analytic review. *International Journal of Psychological Studies, 4*(4), 18–26, www.ccsenet.org/journal/index.php/ijps/article/view/18906/14332 Retrieved 15 December 2014.

Murphy, D. (2019). Understanding and solving the diversity crisis in clinical psychology selection. Paper presented at the Group of Trainers in Clinical Psychology Annual Conference. Liverpool, 4-6 November.

Newnes, C. (2019). *A critical A-Z of electroshock.* Steyning: Real Press.

Newnes, C. (2018) The state and state(us) of clinical psychology. *Clinical Psychology Forum, 309,* 39–45.

Newnes, C. (2016). *Inscription, diagnosis, deception and the mental health: How psy governs us all.* Basingstoke: Palgrave Macmillan.

Nobles, W. (2006). *Seeking the sakhu: Foundational writings for an African psychology.* Chicago, IL: Third World Press.

Parham, T. A. (Ed.) (2002). *Counselling persons of African descent: Raising the bar of practitioner competence.* Thousand Oaks, CA: Sage.

Parry-Jones, W. L. (1972). *The trade in lunacy: A study of private madhouses in England in the eighteenth and nineteenth centuries.* London: Routledge & Kegan Paul.

Patel, N., Bennett, E., Dennis, M., Dosanjh, N., Mahtani, A., Miller, A., & Nadirshaw, Z. (Eds.). (2000). *Clinical psychology, 'race' and culture: A training manual.* Leicester: British Psychological Society.

Ryle, J. (2020). *White privilege: How to be part of the solution.* London: Jessica Kingsley Publishers.

Sengar, K. S. (2019) Suicide: An unresolved enigma. Editorial. *Indian Journal of Clinical Psychology 46*(1), 1–4.

Shockley, W. (1971). Models, mathematics, and the moral obligation to diagnose the origin of Negro IQ deficits. *Review of Educational Research, 41*(4), 369–377. https://doi.org/10.3102/00346543041004369

Terman, L. M. (1930). Autobiography of Lewis M. Terman. In C. Murchison (Ed.). *History of Psychology in Autobiography* (vol. 2, pp. 297–331). Worcester, MA: Clark University Press.

Turpin, G., & Coleman, G. (2010). *Clinical psychology and diversity: Progress and continuing challenges.* Leicester: British Psychological Society.

Turpin, G., & Fensom, P. (2004). *Widening access within undergraduate psychology education and its implications for professional psychology: Gender, disability and ethnic diversity* (pp. 1–80). Leicester: British Psychological Society.

York, K. (2020). BAME representation and psychology. *The Psychologist, 33,* 4.

Zborowski, M., & Herzog, E. (1995). *Life is with people: The culture of the shtetl* New York: Schocken Books.

Chapter 2

Invisible anti-semitism in psychology

Kate Miriam Loewenthal

Summary

Although Suman Fernando has recently and eloquently documented institutional racism in psychiatry and clinical psychology, this has been from the perspective of contemporary Black history. This chapter looks at another form of racism – anti-semitism, particularly invisible anti-semitism. I will look first at definitions of anti-semitism, and the question whether it is on the increase. Turning to psychology I will offer some experiences from my life in psychology, and from the experiences of others, including experiences in universities in general, and some evidence from the history of psychology. Both visible and invisible anti-semitism will be described. One central issue is the 'invisibility' of Jewishness, the difficulty of identifying Jews as such, and the consequences of this, including the wish of many Jews for their Jewishness to be invisible.

Definitions of anti-semitism

Here are some definitions of anti-semitism, from four different sources. The definitions generally incorporate negative beliefs about Jews and may incorporate hostile action.

- Anti-semite: 'A person who is hostile to or prejudiced against Jews.' (Oxford Dictionaries, accessed March 2017)
- 'Antisemitism is a certain perception of Jews, which may be expressed as hatred toward Jews. Rhetorical and physical manifestations of anti-semitism are directed toward Jewish or non-Jewish individuals and/or their property, toward Jewish community institutions and religious facilities.' (International Holocaust Remembrance Alliance (IHRA) May 2016, accessed March 2017)
- 'The government is to formally adopt a definition of what constitutes antisemitism (above), which includes over-sweeping condemnation of Israel i.e., anti-Israel views are formally recognised as anti-semitic' (www.businessinsider.com/britain-new-anti-semitism-definition-2016-12, accessed March 2017)

- 'The belief or behaviour hostile toward Jews just because they are Jewish. It may take the form of religious teachings that proclaim the inferiority of Jews, for instance, or political efforts to isolate, oppress, or otherwise injure them. It may also include prejudiced or stereotyped views about Jews.' (ADL Anti-Defamation League, accessed March 2017)

A fascinating social-psychological perspective summarised by Cuddy (e.g. Cuddy et al., 2008) suggests that there are two dimensions of prejudice; warmth and competence. Jews (and other socioeconomically successful minorities) are seen as competent but not warm: respected but not liked. This is envious prejudice. As well as Jews, other targets include the Tutsi, and the Chinese. In stable conditions, competence is valued. When times are hard, envy and dislike rise to the fore, can be very sudden and the minority group 'deserve to suffer and die'.

Is anti-semitism on the increase?

Overwhelmingly, the consensual answer is yes (see e.g. Loewenthal, 2017). As we shall see, sometimes it is clearly visible, sometimes politely unacknowledged and invisible. Here are examples from many media reports.

This example is from an article by the then NUS (National Union of Students) president Megan Dunn (Huffington Post, 3 November 2016):

> a poster saying 'Hitler was right' on campus, and people tweeting … to say that Jewish people should be 'popped back in the oven' … graphics …which call Jews 'Zionist racist scum' and suggests the Holocaust was 'invented'. The people who write blogs that 9/11 was an 'insurance scam' by 'a secret Jewish network'. Those who write on Facebook that 'Adolf and Co should have finished the job properly', pose questions like 'why stop at 6 million?' and the artists who depict Jews as thieves with big noses.

July 2018, leading Jewish newspapers described the UK Labour party as an 'existential threat to Jewish life in this country'. The party leader Jeremy Corbyn was accused of being a racist and an anti-semite. This perception of Corbyn's anti-semitism persisted amidst growing concern, resulting in the defection of several Labour MPs (members of parliament) from the Labour party, explicitly on the grounds of their concerns over the anti-semitism issue. The vast majority of Labour MPs however remained within the party. An article in the *New Stateman* offered a guide to contemporary anti-semitism. The article argued that current anti-semitic conspiracy theories – regarding both left and right-wing anti-semitism – all suggest that *undue influence is wielded by Jews covertly acting in concert with one another.* Often manifested in a fervent loathing of Israel, alongside a claim that Israel is imperialist, that anti-Zionism is not anti-semitism, often coupled with the horrendously ironic accusation that Israel is 'Nazi scum'. The International Holocaust Remembrance Alliance's definition of anti-semitism (accepted by governments and mainstream politicial parties throughout the democratic world) has been rewritten by the UK Labour party. According to this it is NOT anti-semitic to claim that Jews are Nazis or Nazi sympathisers; (and not anti-semitic to claim) that they are conspirators in thrall to Israel … on the basis of their race.

Apart from descriptive media material offering vivid examples of contemporary anti-semitism, the Institute for Jewish Policy research (Boyd, 2018) offers an array of convincing figures from a survey of over 16,000 (mainly Western) European Jews. The survey was conducted for the EU (European Union) Agency for Fundamental Rights (FRA). Findings include:

- Almost 90% of respondents across all countries surveyed say they feel *that levels of anti-semitism have increased* in their country over the past five years, with the highest proportions found in France, Poland, Belgium and Germany.
- The online environment, particularly social media, is most noxious.
- Comparisons (made where possible) with 2012 data: concerns about the *levels of online anti-semitism have increased* over the past five years.
- Other arenas also regarded as particularly problematic across Europe were the street, in the media and in political life.
- The ideas that European Jews are most likely to consider anti-semitic include Holocaust denial and minimisation, and *claims that Jews deliberately exploit Holocaust victimhood* for their own purposes.
- The anti-semitic ideas that European Jews are most likely to encounter include comparisons between Israelis and Nazis and contentions that Jews have too much power in their country. Half (51%) report that they have heard non-Jewish people express the former idea in the past 12 months, and 43% the latter.
- 28% of Jews surveyed say that they have experienced some form of anti-semitic harassment in the past 12 months.

Anti-semitism in psychology

Published descriptive and quantitative evidence suggests that anti-semitism is on the rise. What has been happening in psychology?

What follow are some personal experiences from my life in psychology, chiefly in academia. I began to study psychology in 1960 and was appointed to a full-time academic post in 1966. I remained in full-time academic psychology until 2004, when I retired and began to work part-time: teaching, writing, editorial work, speaking and clinical work.

I was bewildered by academic psychology's failure to take psychodynamic psychology seriously. It was accused of being 'unscientific', but psychology students were seldom given opportunities to find out what it involved. I and a colleague wished to start an undergraduate course in which theory, practice and evidence were presented. At the meeting to discuss this course proposal, the head of the psychology department came up with the fairly famous stereotype: psychoanalysts are Jewish doctors who can't bear the sight of blood. Witty? Perhaps. True? What is the evidence? Anti-semitic? Very possibly – Jewish doctors are not real doctors, squeamish, not tough enough to do the real job. And a good example of invisible, unacknowledged anti-semitism.

Israel under constant siege, with conscription of almost every adult male, had and has a high proportion of fatherless children. On one occasion I was collecting for Jewish war orphans among psychology academics. One of them wanted to know why I wasn't (also) collecting for Palestinian war orphans. Invisible, unacknowledged anti-semitism? I said that I would be happy to donate to a collection for Palestinian war orphans – I asked if this colleague wanted to start collecting. (They did not start collecting.)

Unfortunately I have repressed the details of the exact words spoken in the next example. I entered the senior common room of a university at which I was giving a guest lecture. The room was very peaceful mid-afternoon, with only two male academics sitting on a comfortable sofa. I sat quietly in a cosy arm-chair with my back to the two, probably not noticeable. But I could hear that they were gossiping about a Jewish colleague, sniggering about his unfortunate Jewish traits. It was an experience in which my blood ran pretty cold – they were speaking as if they believed they were unheard (and invisible?), and I had never previously heard such explicit anti-semitism live.

My next example was, I believe, the result of my being a strictly orthodox Jewish woman, committed to having many children. I would like to explain here that, in order not to provoke anti-semitism, I did the same hours of teaching as my colleagues in the years when I gave birth, and tried to ensure that no colleagues shouldered any extra burdens for me in periods when I was giving birth. I tried (and I think succeeded) to keep up a good output of research articles, and succeeded in generating good research income – these indices of academic productivity compared favourably with those of colleagues but I was disappointed that I did not always gain promotion when I could see that colleagues with similar achievements were being promoted. In fact my head of department said explicitly 'You will ruin your career by having so many children'. This was even though the evidence showed that I was as productive (or more productive) of good work as colleagues with smaller families or no children.

I turn now to some examples involving academic administration, in which covert anti-semitism could sometimes be experienced behind the mask of bureaucratically governed correct procedure.

It is common practice for university examinations to be conducted in the early summer, and further examinations may be held at other times. Difficulties for observant Jewish students are caused when early summer examinations may be timetabled on the festival of Shavuot. Examinations late in the summer – for example resitting an early summer examination – may clash with the Jewish autumn festivals, particularly the New Year. I experienced a notable absence of anti-semitism when the registrar of my university asked if I could provide the dates of Jewish festivals every year, so that the authorities could avoid timetabling examinations on those days. But other examples brought to my attention frequently involved the summer examinations, and some universities were not helpful. It was suggested to university authorities that observant Jewish students might be allowed to sit the examination after the festival, at a religiously permitted time, with offers to ensure there had been no access to the examination questions. Some universities and examining boards were willing to go along with such suggestions, displaying both goodwill and effort to accommodate, other administrators were less helpful, with an undercurrent of hostility. On one occasion it was suggested that if students chose not to sit an examination they could take the appropriate consequences of this choice, and fail. Some university authorities would argue that they would have to make similar concessions to students from other faith traditions. These arguments were also applied when orthodox Jewish students experienced difficulties in attending Friday afternoon classes in winter, when the Sabbath begins (in Northern latitudes) very early. I would point out that in Islam, for example, there are no restrictions on activities such as using motorised transport or writing on the holy day of the week, provided prayer obligations were fulfilled. This seemed to leave Jewish supplicants with the feeling that they were asking for unreasonable favours. One orthodox Jewish student arriving from overseas had felt obliged to agree to stay in the university hall of residence: he was provided with an electronic key for his room. Such a key cannot be used on the Sabbath. A complete stranger in town, he spent the entire Friday night and Saturday wandering around without shelter or food, and when he asked for help in getting his door open the following week (it is religiously permitted to seek such help) his request was declined on the grounds that this was an unreasonable burden on the university's services. The problem was resolved by the intervention of a senior figure in the university who was orthodox Jewish himself, but I fear the problem left a trail of bad feeling.

In psychology and psychiatry, the area is littered with stereotypes, in which the concealment or blatancy of anti-semitism varies.

Much of my research has focused on distress in the Jewish community. When I meet someone at a conference and they discover I am speaking on this topic, a common response is: Ah, orthodox Jews, there must be a lot of OCD (obsessive compulsive disorder). In fact the evidence is not at all conclusive. The stereotype is that, with all those strict rules governing every detail – for example tying the right shoelaces after the left – religious practitioners become obsessionally focused on details. In practice, those diagnosed with OCD can be pretty choosy. Sufferers do not focus on every detail of everything; albeit the selectivity is not consciously operated. Someone may organise their french fries in order of size, but not their books. They may wash their hands frequently and rigorously, but not their feet. Chris Lewis' review (1999) made sense to me – religiosity is associated with scrupulosity, but not with high levels of obsessionality. Several studies show no association between levels of religiosity and OCD among Jews and, indeed, in other faith traditions. It has been concluded that religious ritual is an arena for the expression of OCD, but not a causal factor (e.g. Greenberg & Wiztum, 2001; Zohar et al., 2005; Al-Solaim & Loewenthal, 2011).

Here is another stereotype – based on research that was fed to me as an undergraduate in the 1960s – to the effects that children from large families were less intelligent and achieved less than children from small families. This research has been done in different cultural settings to those inhabited by Jews, but nevertheless gave rise to the idea that children in large families would suffer deprivation due to the dilution of resources (e.g. Downey, 1995). This idea was expressed to me by some colleagues as a possibility for orthodox Jewish families, where average family size was much larger than the norm in Western society, but the research on this topic has been very limited. One conclusion has been that the lack of (clear detrimental) effect of family size on educational attainment in Jews and others (Shavit & Pierce, 1991) is an effect of the positive value placed on family size in the Jewish community, coupled with the cohesion of the Jewish community, its support for nuclear families, and its practice of extended hours of schooling.

Another suggestion about family size is that larger families are more dysfunctional than smaller families, and the children of larger families are therefore more likely to show behavioural and emotional disturbances. In fact family size does not relate to behaviour disturbance in Jewish children (Lindsey et al., 2003; Frosh et al., 2005).

There are a number of ideas about Jews and mental health. I have already mentioned the OCD stereotype. Other suggestions have been that Jews are prone to 'mood disorders', sometimes implying a possible diagnosis of bipolar disorder. Research on the genetic susceptibility of Jews to bipolar disorders and schizophrenia has produced inconsistent findings (e.g. Fallin et al., 2004).

With regard to mood disorders, Jewish men in the USA were reported to be more likely be diagnosed with depression than men in other religious-cultural groups: Levav et al. (1997) reported that

> Jews had a 1:1 female-to-male ratio for major depression, in contrast to the other religious groups, which approached the universal 2:1 ratio. Rates of alcohol abuse/dependence were inversely related to rates of major depression. The results support only in part the earlier reports that Jews have higher rates of major depression. The equal gender distribution of major depression among Jews may be associated with the lower rate of alcoholism among Jewish males.

Loewenthal et al (1995; 2003) supported these results and conclusions: orthodox Jewish men are more susceptible to depression than men from other groups, probably at least partly the result of not using alcohol to cope with low mood. This rather finicky detailed explanation seldom rises to the surface – the stereotype remains: 'Jews are prone to mood disorders.'

What other Jewish mental health stereotypes have I come across? The internet may help to disseminate mental health stereotypes, and this covers almost everything! And probably based on just one case: 'I am an Ashkenazi Jew. Ashkenazi Jews are often anxious. We can also be high-strung, irritable, obsessive, depressive, creative and brilliant – think Woody Allen.' (recipistsdiary.com/2016/11/05/admd-ashkenazi, 9 March 2019). The wording is cautious – 'are often', 'can also be', but the stereotypes are there. Research has shown little or no truth in these and other stereotypes, but they can be persistent, and may interfere with the help that Jews may receive from mental health professionals.

In an eloquent chapter in a book on Jewish women in psychotherapy, Evelyn Beck (1991) argues that the stereotype of the JAP (Jewish American Princess) deals women a double blow: anti-semitic and misogynist. The traditional anti-semitic sterotype of the Jew, as in Shakespeare's Shylock, is manipulative, calculating and avaricious, materialistic, sexually perverse and ugly (hook-nosed). The JAP is accused of all these characteristics, with a misogynist twist: manipulative of men, calculating and avaricious in getting men's money, materialistically focused on appearance and possessions, sexually perverse and ugly – she needs or has had a 'nose job'. Beck describes a number of incidents in which the JAP is humiliated, stigmatised and threatened with annihilation – for example, campus t-shirts saying 'slap-a-JAP'.

Campus anti-semitism has a long history. In the history of psychology, Winston (1998) provided an astonishing depiction of the activities of the distinguished Harvard professor of psychology, E. G. Boring. In a paper evocatively titled 'The defects of his race: E. G. Boring and Antisemitism in American Psychology, 1923–1953', Winston describes how from the 1920s to the 1950s, Boring wrote letters of reference for Jewish students and colleagues in which he followed the common practice – seen as an obligation – of identifying them as Jews and assessing whether they showed the 'objectionable traits' thought to characterise Jews. The objectionable traits seemed to be particularly those of personality rather than of academic ability. This is discussed in relation to the increasing anti-semitism of the interwar period. Winston's article has specific reference to Abraham A. Roback and Kurt Lewin. In Roback's case, the 'defect' of Jewishness was thought to explain his 'undesirable personality' – he unlike most others was very committed to Yiddish and Jewish organisations, and to emphasising the positive role of Jews in academic psychology. With Lewin, personal charm mitigated the 'defect' of Jewishness. Here are some samples of Boring's references:

> You would get a good and enthusiastic worker in X … but I most emphatically do not recommend him, because he has some of the personal unpleasantnesses that are usually associated with Jews.
>
> Y is a Jew, and his inferiority sometimes expresses itself in aggression.
>
> [And a more favourable] Z is a Jew but doesn't show it much.

After World War II the obligations to identify Jews lessened, for various reasons, including (possibly) increased assimilation and secularisation. Unfortunately nowadays, there is widespread agreement about the resurgence of anti-semitism. And this is something with a long, long historical legacy.

Invisibility

The talk on which this chapter is based was entitled 'Invisible anti-semitism in psychology'. Craig Newnes organised the symposium in which the talk was included, and mentioned the issue of administrators organising events on Jewish festivals, which many Jews would not be willing or able to attend – either because, being orthodox, they would not break Jewish law which forbids activities such as using vehicles for travel and writing. Or because as traditional Jews they would not wish to spend important festivals such as the New Year or Yom Kippur (Day of Repentance) occupied with workaday matters. Nevertheless this clash of religious and secular obligations may not be deliberately anti-semitic, and is not usually even noticeable and visible as causing problems for Jews. Invisible anti-semitism again.

This 'invisibility' of anti-semitism invites me to examine something which may be related – the 'invisibility' of Jewishness. This issue was highlighted for me some years ago by an Irish friend (Gerard Leavey): he thought there was something extra scary for the majority culture in having to deal with a minority that normally doesn't look obviously different (such as Irish or Jewish). It can be very difficult to identify Jews or Irish, or other white minorities as such. Boring in the 1930–50 period often complained how hard it was to identify whether someone was Jewish, though he felt he was expected to explain the extent to which Jewish candidates for jobs in psychology showed the 'defects of their race'.

Weiss (2014) asks in 'More than meets the eye', how anti-semitism differs from forms of racism based on physical appearance. Or does this prejudice have to be based on purported physical appearance? Nazis claimed that Jews had an unsightly appearance. But they were apparently so difficult to identify that they were required to be identified with a yellow star. Frazier Glenn Cross in the USA claimed that Jews were 'swarthy, hairy, bow-legged, beady-eyed, parasitic midgets'. He drove to Jewish institutions in Kansas City and murdered three people he believed to be Jewish (they were two Methodists and a Catholic).

Many Jews wish their Jewishness to be invisible. A young Jewish boy in a play centre wished to remove his *yarmulke* (religious head covering) as it made him different from everybody else. A woman learning BSL (British Sign Language) was upset to learn that the sign for 'Jew' denoted a beard. For months afterwards she experienced somatic signs of distress when thinking of this. More subtly, a non-Jewish student of Jewish Studies at University College London, Isobel Carter, recently wrote of frequent questions addressed to anyone Jewish (or with Jewish interests). They might be asked questions especially regarding Israel: 'So what do you think of the Arab-Israel conflict?' 'Have you met any

Palestinians?' and many questions about the actions of the Israeli government. She concludes 'It makes them uncomfortable to be Jewish.'

Fisher (2004) asked why distinguished Jewish psychoanalysts after World War II muted their left-wing and socialist political tendencies once they arrived in America, taking a turn against politics. Fisher noted a 'pronounced ambivalence of this generation of Jewish analysts and intellectuals against their own Jewish backgrounds and sense of themselves as Jews'. Fisher sees their exploration of Jewish psychology as a disguised form of racism.

A non-Jewish clinical psychologist described an orthodox Jewish colleague 'with his beard and black hat and strings (*Tsitzis*) … we were all very proud of him'. Another colleague, conversely, described feeling bewildered by a (non-orthodox) Jewish colleague who chose bacon for breakfast.

I concluded from this invisibility that, generally, Jewishness can indeed be difficult to detect. Jews may wish to conceal their Jewishness. But at least some non-Jews may prefer clear Jewish identification. The invisibility of Jewishness creates suspicion and feeds invisible anti-semitism.

Conclusion

This chapter focused on invisible anti-semitism in psychology, and in the academic and clinical worlds in general. This anti-semitism is not strictly invisible, it is simply not explicit or acknowledged. I mention a number of examples, many from personal experience, scattered across the last century. I also offer some observations and comments on the invisibility of Jewishness, and the ways in which this may contribute to anti-semitism in academia and elsewhere.

References

Al-Solaim, L., & Loewenthal, K. M. (2011). Religion and obsessive-compulsive disorder (OCD) among young Muslim women in Saudi Arabia. *Mental Health, Religion and Culture, 14*, 169–182. DOI:https://doi.org/10.1080/13674676.2010.544868

Beck, E. T. (1991). Therapy's double dilemma: Anti-semitism and misogyny. In R. J. Siegel & E. Cole (Eds.). *Jewish women in therapy: Seen but not heard* (pp. 19–30). New York: Harrington Park Press.

Boyd, J. (2018). *Reflections on the European Union Agency for Fundamental Rights (FRA) survey of Jewish people's experiences and perceptions of antisemitism*. London: Institute of Jewish Policy Research.

Carter, I. (2018). No, I do not have a thing for Jews. *HJS (The University College London Department of Jewish and Hebrew Studies Journal)*, December, 7–9.

Cuddy, A. J. C., Fiske, S. T., & Glick, P. (2008). Warmth and competence as universal dimensions of social perception: The stereotype content model and the BIAS Map. *Advances in Experimental Social Psychology, 40*, 62–137. DOI: 10.1016/S0065-2601(07)00002-0

Downey, D. (1995). When bigger is not better: Family size, parental resources, and children's educational performance. *American Sociological Review, 60*(5), 746. DOI: 10.2307/2096320

Fallin, M. D., Lasseter, V. K., Wolyniec, P. S., et al. (2004). Genomewide linkage scan for bipolar-disorder susceptibility loci among Ashkenazi Jewish families. *American Journal of Human Genetics*, *75*(2), 204–219. DOI: https://doi.org/10.1086/422474

Fernando, S. (2017). *Institutional racism in psychiatry and clinical psychology: Race matters in mental health* (Contemporary Black History). London: Palgrave Macmillan.

Fisher, D. J. (2004). Towards a psychoanalytic understanding of Fascism and anti-Semitism: Perceptions from the 1940s. *Psychoanalysis and History*, *6*(1), 57–74. DOI: https://doi.org/10.3366/pah.2004.6.1.57

Frosh, S., Loewenthal, K. M., Lindsey, C., & Spitzer, E. (2005). Prevalence of emotional and behavioural disorders among strictly orthodox Jewish children in London. *Clinical Child Psychology and Psychiatry, 10,* 351–368. DOI: https://doi.org/10.1177/1359104505053754

Greenberg, D., & Witztum, E. (2001). *Sanity and sanctity: Mental health work among the ultra-orthodox in Jerusalem.* New Haven, CT, and London: Yale University Press. DOI: 10.12987/yale/9780300071917.001.0001

Levav, I., Kohn, R. Golding, J., & Weismann, M. M. (1997). Vulnerability of Jews to affective disorders. *American Journal of Psychiatry, 154*, 941–947. DOI: 10.1176/ajp.154.7.941

Lindsey, C., Frosh, S., Loewenthal, K. M., & Spitzer, E. (2003). Prevalence of emotional and behavioural disorders among strictly orthodox Jewish pre-school children in London. *Clinical Child Psychology and Psychiatry, 8*, 459–472. DOI: https://doi.org/10.1177/13591045030084004

Loewenthal, K. M. (2017). Anti-semitism and its mental health effects. Royal College of Psychiatry, Spirituality & Psychiatry Special Interest Group Conference: Stigma, discrimination and spirituality. London, April.

Loewenthal, K. M., Goldblatt, V., Gorton, T., et al. (1995). Gender and depression in Anglo-Jewry. *Psychological Medicine, 25*, 1051–1063. DOI: 10.1017/S0033291700037545

Loewenthal, K. M., MacLeod, A. K., Cook, S., et al. (2003). Beliefs about alcohol among UK Jews and Protestants: Do they fit the alcohol-depression hypothesis? *Social Psychiatry and Psychiatric Epidemiology*, *38,* 122–127. DOI: 10.1007/s00127-003-0609-4

McInnis, E. (2002). Institutional racism in the NHS and clinical psychology. *Journal of Critical Psychology, Counselling and Psychotherapy*, Autumn, 164–170.

Shavit, Y., & Pierce, J. L. (1991). Sibship size and educational attainment in nuclear and extended families: Arabs and Jews in Israel. *American Sociological Review*, *56*(30), 321–330. DOI: https://doi.org/10.2307/2096107

Weiss, D. (2014). Anti-semitism: More than meets the eye. Posted 28 April 2014. Accessed 12 May 2019. https://blogs.timesofisrael.com/anti-semitism-more-than-meets-the-eye/

Winston, A. S. (1998). The defects of his race: E. G. Boring and antisemitism in American psychology, 1923–1953. *History of Psychology*, *1*(1), 27–51. http://dx.doi.org/10.1037/1093-4510.1.1.27

Zohar, A. H., Goldman, E., Calamary, R., and Mashiah, M. (2005). Religiosity and obsessive–compulsive behavior in Israeli Jews. *Behaviour Research and Therapy, 43*(7), 857–868. https://doi.org/10.1016/j.brat.2004.06.009

Chapter 3

The global system of white supremacy within UK clinical psychology

An African psychology perspective

Erica Mapule McInnis

Summary

This chapter analyses UK institutional racism in clinical psychology from an African psychology perspective while appreciating others. Issues are relevant to other branches of psychology. It suggests the term 'global system of White supremacy' rather than racism and considers a satirical future such a system may be defending against. It further suggests institutional racism has an added new wave of strategies from direct government such as Brexit and the Windrush scandal (which is proposed better termed a Maafa, a Kiswahili term for great disaster). Such policies produce a pervasive psychology climate which excels in inducing fear, interrupting progress, traumatising and propagandising as inferior world majority people. Underlying psychological mechanisms such as implicit bias against Black people and favouritism towards White people are argued to impact clinical psychologists before, during and after training, alongside issues such as class and disability. The focus of McInnis (2002) is reflected upon with additional thinking for resilience, recovery and renewal from the paradigm of African psychology. This is in case the tactics change but the game remains the same. The aim is to imagine a clinical psychology anew.

Let us look to where we could be if the past was different. The satirical year is 2040.

- Several African countries send aid to the UK post Brexit (a referendum vote in 2016 for Britain to leave the European Union).
- No longer needing to fund projects in African countries, the charity Comic Relief funds what was the NHS (National Health Service).
- The UK pays reparations rather than aid to the continent of Africa due to the transatlantic slave trade.
- African psychology is standard as both a university module and course with appropriate accreditation from supporting regulating bodies and trade unions.
- Children and adults are taught African psychology as one of several paradigms for emotional wellness and happiness.

- Teaching Kemetic[1] origins of psychology are standard (Akbar, 1994) and decolonising the curriculum is interwoven throughout courses and an integral part of professional training bodies.
- Progressive university psychology training courses now hold one-day seminars to add Eurocentric thinking to an African-based curriculum.
- There is a range of tools to incorporate African psychology into clinical work, supervision and research.
- Health services are reclassified as healing and transformation services. As appropriate they offer multidimensional and holistic healing such as exercise, nutrition, mindfulness, traditional healing, flow and high vibrational living strategies (Craig, 2013; Csikszentmihalyi, 2002; Nobles, 2006).
- Children and young people are taught to General Certificate of Secondary Education (GCSE) level about the British empire and different forms of colonialism from the perspective of interruption to the progress of the doctor, engineer, architect and leader enslaved.

Could this satirical future be too woke[2] for some people?

Where are we now?

Let's turn the clock back to when I wrote an article (McInnis, 2002) on institutional racism in the NHS and clinical psychology. This was post the McPherson report (McPherson, 1999), a report produced following the UK murder of Black teenager Stephen Lawrence which highlighted racism at various levels in the police force. Hence, the atmosphere was ripe for analysis of institutional racism in other institutions.

Nearly 20 years later, the psychology of racism at an institutional level (Fernando, 2017) appears to have been joined by 'Big Brother'[3] at the governmental level. For example, government policies and a state enforced 'hostile environment' towards anyone who may appear foreign contributed to the Windrush scandal. The latter saw a plethora of law-abiding British citizens (some of whom served or contributed to 'rebuilding' the UK post war), wrongly classified as illegal immigrants. This led to threats and deportation, emotional turmoil, constant fear with self-removal by some, loss of homes, separation of families, loss of employment, loss of access to health and social care services and in some cases early death (Gentleman, 2019; Vernon, 2019).

This was a major blow to the psychological well-being of families and communities as elders in Black[4] cultures are often keepers of wisdom and integral to child rearing in extended family structures (Boyd-Franklin, 2006; Boyd-Franklin, 1989; Karenga, 2010). Fighting deportation of an elder can drain a family's resources both emotionally and financially. This was and is a great disaster for both Black and White communities as many UK families are multiracial (McInnis & Moukam, 2013). The term Maafa[5] (Great Disaster to Black people; Ani, 1997a) is applicable to this disaster as a continuation of injustice based upon racial differences.

Race-based hostility is in UK social and recreational settings (Kick It Out, 2019; Cleland & Cashmore 2013) and fundamentally global, as demonstrated by the Black Lives Matter movement. The latter publicised Black people's experience of dehumanising police brutality and failures of the criminal justice system to protect them (Heatherton & Camp, 2016). Reporting such events has the potential to further traumatise and invoke fear, particularly when repeatedly shared on social media (Segundo, 2017). When such traumas mainly affect Black people, are UK psychological therapy services equipped with something other than a Eurocentric response? Furthermore, would individuals affected meet referral criteria set by providers of therapy services, given many will have coexisting resilience (Keyes, 2009)?

Such incidents appear set to continue. As leaders of countries increasingly become overt in their racism or White nationalism, the question is asked, do such leaders represent their followers or inspire them (*The Guardian*, 2019; *Washington Post*, 2018)? According to Reddie (2019) xenophobia is now a part of UK culture. Xenophobia is like racism, but instead of fearing or distrusting people predominantly because of the colour of their skin, fear or distrust is because of their nationality, or that they seem foreign. I argue deep pigmentation of skin can arouse suspicion of foreign status whether applicable or not.

How does racism manifest then and now?

Institutional racism is the existence of historical and current policies, laws and practices that provide worse treatment or access to goods, services and opportunities for certain racial groups. In short, society is structured so that people of the highest skin pigmentation (darker in complexion) have worse experiences, although the impact can vary depending upon coping, resilience and other factors (Eddo-Lodge, 2017). As this is a global phenomenon, it is argued that it is better defined by its recipients as a 'global system of White Supremacy'[6] (Fuller, 2016).

Workplace experiences

From reports from others and my own, Black people too frequently become troubled individuals in troubled workplace institutions (Obholzer & Roberts, 2009). Such institutions either unconsciously or consciously select a person to voice or process a grievance. This is often to 'work through' or voice on behalf of a group difficult, disowned and anxiety-provoking aspects of the workplace. It is argued Black people are frequently selected for this task, first, due to favouritism to White people and secondly, as they have a history of doing the work others do not want (Eddo-Lodge 2017). Indeed, they often find themselves with limited options due to circumstances. For example, 'In Acute, PCT [Primary Care Trust], Mental Health and Learning Disability and Care trusts, BME staff were significantly over-represented in disciplinary proceedings'

(Archibong & Darr, 2010). Furthermore, Black and Minority Ethnic (BME) staff disproportionately experience bullying and harassment (Lintern, 2017). Although recommendations are in place which may improve the situation, over-representation in disciplinary proceedings often contributes to a scarcity of effective role models for Black communities.

I am informed of situations where it seemed consciously or unconsciously engineered for members of different protected groups (Equality Act, 2010)[7] to come into conflict with each other. The result can be members of protected groups working through unconscious feelings present in the group on behalf of the wider group. This occurrence is usually stirred by the emotionally challenging nature of the task to be done (Halton, 2009). For example, two of the individuals in a group, one individual White and homosexual the other Black and heterosexual, are consciously or unconsciously excluded by the group so left to work together on an impossible or highly difficult task. One view is conflict would result in removal of one protected group member; which results in White, heterosexual, middle-class men (and in the profession of clinical psychology often women) continuing to dominate. Alternatively, both individuals with protected characteristics could struggle with the culture of the other's protected characteristic. A White person with a protected status does not necessarily have compassion around issues of race. Also, I have seen limited workplace training courses on understanding Whiteness (Wood & Patel, 2017), but many diversity courses which primarily aim to help White people understand Black people. Thus, Black people can often be disadvantaged in understanding the cultural context in which they are to thrive. Some support may be available through Black Staff Network groups (Coghill & Kline, 2017) in health settings. However, this can attract Black staff ranging from professionals to non-professionals at varying levels in their career with very different needs. Also, I have heard reports of such networks having been set objectives by an institution in the interest of the institution, with little focus on meeting the support needs of staff.

I've been told of incidents where bullying and harassment policies developed to protect Black and HOMMS (Historically, Oppressed, Marginalised, Minority-status, and/or Stigmatised)[8] people, are used against the very people they are designed to protect. This could be for many reasons such as projection identification where an institution projects onto the Black person, so the Black person becomes a 'sponge' for all the anger, depression and guilt in the situation (Halton 2009). In such situations the institution is often defended against hearing, listening or acknowledging the significance of their role in oppression (Moylan, 2009). So, when a Black person reports inappropriate behaviour from an institution member, that Black person becomes a target for the institution. Such situations can affect the confidence of that Black person. Furthermore, what can start as a conflict between a single White and a Black person, can soon escalate to an unequal struggle by a powerful wounded organisation against a solitary Black person. It would seem reasonable to imply confirmation bias could and would take place in investigation procedures where those in authority consciously or unconsciously both seek and prefer information which confirms an implicit cultural bias against a Black person. This can be based on their preferences, perception of trustworthiness, misperceptions, stereotypes or blatant misunderstandings of Black people and their culture (Cooke, 2018; De Houwer, 2019; Moylan 2009). It is proposed that such cultural bias presents a danger of a self-fulfilling prophecy within investigations where the process of addressing non-existent, exaggerated or unnecessarily targeted issues leads to the development of problems. For instance, Fein (2018) gives the example of job interviewers behaving in a colder interpersonal style towards Black interviewees, leading Black interviewees to behave in a more nervous and awkward style.

> In short, the Whites' racial stereotype and prejudice actually hurt the interview performance of the Black candidates … It seemed to confirm the interviewers' negative stereotype – but this poor performance was caused by the interviewers, not the interviewees.
>
> (Fein, 2018, 20)

Although this may not be the only issue at play, how often does this happen in clinical psychology and the systems clinical psychologists work in?

Fein (2018) goes on to suggest communication of distrust towards Black people reduces their sense of belonging. It leads them to deeply feel that 'people like me do not belong here'. It is argued this may be particularly pronounced for Black psychologists as they rise within a profession that is predominantly White and steeped in racism (Guthrie, 1998; Turpin & Coleman, 2010). Furthermore, Fein (2018) states the esteem of the group a person strongly identifies with (e.g. Black) is important to how they see themselves. Therefore, it is reasonable to expect the police shooting of a Black youth in 2011 which led to riots in multiple UK cities, for a period of time both affected the self-esteem of Black professionals and how they were seen by colleagues. Indeed, I know employees in inner-city local authority buildings being sent home early – such was the threat considered to face staff in such institutions (Mail Online, 2019).

How does racism in the psychology industry affect White people?

White psychologists benefit from White privilege (McIntosh, 2003) which is an invisible package of unearned assets society gives those with White skin regardless of social, political or economic circumstances. These include cultural affirmations of White people's worth; presumed greater social status; and freedom to move, buy, work, play and speak freely. The effects can be seen in professional, educational and personal contexts and imply the right to assume the universality of one's own experiences, marking others as different or exceptional while perceiving oneself as normal. It is my perception that

White psychologists and colleagues are instantly trusted in the workplace due to advantage and favouritism bestowed on Whiteness (DiTomaso, 2015). Whereas Black psychologists often need to prove themselves, and then co-work with colleagues who were initially highly suspicious of them. Stereotypes of doubt can seep into perception of trustworthiness in an area as basic as claiming mileage and other administrative tasks. It can also lead to a barrage of investigations or issues raised, as a team can engage in confirmation bias, seeking information which confirms their biases (DiTomaso, 2015). Time spent managing such negative stereotypes drain energy and can mean Black psychologists often work a 'double shift' to manage such issues. Vance (2001) referred to the term 'psychological taxation' to describe this phenomenon which is part of the burden Black people carry due to racism. Psychologists often write of unease even speaking of such experiences (Adetimole et al., 2005; McInnis, 2002).

The implementation of a system of White supremacy can include use of or coexistence with other forms of oppression due to class, gender and disability (Akala, 2018; Eddo-Lodge, 2017; Jackson-Lowman, 2014; Reeve, 2012). This is to say the combination of being Black, achieving and disability can attract attack. The weapon of choice can be to inconvenience, delay or obstruct reasonable adjustments for a disability, however minor the person's disability. From experiences reported to me, this simultaneity of oppression can delay, confuse, distract, increase the load, derail, hijack, traumatise and distress while also building resilience. It is reasoned by the author that the impetus is to use multiple protected characteristics to sustain the status quo in favour of White people, if Black people are in a position to minimise the effects of oppressive structural barriers (such as disproportionate poverty or deteriorated housing[9]). Indeed, being Black does not provide exemption from structural disablism (Reeve, 2012). For example, I was told of a Black senior professional not being allowed workplace access to a specialty chair provided by occupational health for a diagnosed back condition. In addition to threatening their health and safety, which may be an attempt to further disable, this can give rise to psycho-emotional disablism where the person's well-being and sense of self are adversely affected by their ill treatment (Reeve, 2012).

Provision of support to cope with a simultaneity of oppression can present further issues. I am aware from both my own experience and that of others, many Black and White allies, sensitive to issues of race, reported to be working class. Then, class can become a tension between middle-class Black psychologists and Black or White allies. Allies likely have implicit biases about characteristics such as class, gender, disability, sexuality, culture and family structure (Daiches, 2010; De Houwer, 2019). So, developing a good supportive supervisory or managerial match for Black psychologists as they grow can be an additional struggle due to the range of implicit biases. What is implicit bias? According to De Houwer (2019) implicit bias refers to unconscious negative thinking about a particular group of people learned from mental associations and social conditioning, which lead to negative behaviours towards members of that group. A criticism of such definitions is that they can stimulate lack of responsibility for implicit biases held, with the argument they are unconscious.

Whether intentional or not, implicit bias that Black British are inferior can lead to assumptions that Black people are untrustworthy, lying, shirking on the job and likely to be aggressive. Such experiences and additional struggles can take place at various stages, such as prior to clinical psychology training, during and when qualified (Guilaine, 2014; Odusanya, 2016; Turpin & Coleman, 2010). From my experience and those told to me, this can manifest in workplace team meetings with Black British psychologists needing to demonstrate their point more than others, lacking support and respect, having their work more scrutinised, and rarely receiving feedback that they are good enough. This is not to say such treatment is constant or that they lack opportunities, however a backlash can sometimes outweigh any support. Indeed, searching for credibility and assumptions of not being the psychologist in the room were themes found in qualitative research by Odusanya (2016). I recall situations when male, White trainee clinical psychologists were assumed to be qualified, and I as a Black woman assumed to be the unqualified trainee. This could be for a number of reasons, including race. Reddie (2003) discusses the concept of 'hierarchy of credibility', a ranking system of whose accounts are believed, which has Black women at the bottom.

It would seem implicit bias impacts clinical psychology in varied ways (Vara & Patel, 2012; Dennis & Aitken, 2012; Sue et al., 2007). Turpin & Coleman (2010) suggest some progress regarding potential inequalities within the application process and in raising the awareness of clinical psychology as a profession to Black people. However, they note much room for improvement. Regarding clinical psychology training, Adetimole et al (2005) offer insight on their experience.

> We did not want to be misunderstood as betraying our course, peers and tutors, as some of them were supportive. As Black people we often have to be very careful about how we talk about our experiences, because of our hyperawareness of other people's anxieties, feelings of guilt, anger or suspiciousness towards us. (Adetimole et al., 2005, 11)

There is fear that if they voice concerns and expose issues they would be targeted by a profession arguably defensive or struggling with cultural diversity (Turpin & Coleman, 2010). What is described seems an example of the concept of White fragility. This is where, in various settings, White people come to expect racial comfort, lowering their ability to tolerate racial stress (e.g. Black people voicing the issue of race). Even a minimum amount of conversing about such issues becomes intolerable, triggering a range of defensive moves such as anger, fear, and guilt, and behaviours such as argumentation, silence and leaving the stress-inducing situation (DiAngelo, 2011). It's as if Black people intermittently have access to rights and privileges only if they make White people feel comfortable in their Whiteness. I've heard workplace examples where obscure nebulous parts of policies are applied disproportionately to Black people, which tire, challenge or just frustrate the Black person. This often occurs at crucial times in careers when progress is going well, or exams are final.

I also observed either withdrawal or slowing of labour by members of the workforce when a Black person is in a position of leadership. The aim seems to be to frustrate attempts by Black leaders. This is compounded by new employment practices such as a temporary workforce for specific projects on short-term contracts (if contracted) and movement around different worksites. From conversations I've had with many, such initiatives seem to negatively affect Black people most. At a spiritual level it can feel reminiscent of being repeatedly sold and passed to other plantations, regardless of one's competence.

Although there are benefits of an agile workforce, such initiatives often remove the emotional secure base from which an employee can feel safe and thrive, reduces access to 'on the job' emotional and practical support, and interrupts the capacity to build competence and flow experiences (Bowlby, 1988; Csikszentmihalyi, 2002). It can seem as if a Black person is just moved around until they feel fed-up, spiritually broken and leave (physically or mentally). Even when some institutions have diversity strategies in place, they can be misapplied or misunderstood as oppression of White people and result in engendering far-right White nationalism. Thus, the status quo does not change. Indeed, fear from some White people of oppression seems very misplaced, as Post and DiTomaso (2018) suggest it is 'favouritism to White people which impacts greatest' against Black people. Given this key finding, will there be a time when monitoring of institutions considers favouritism to White people, not only discrimination against Black people?

Implicit bias can prevail even when there is a Black supervisor and White supervisee. Implicit bias can lead a White supervisee to perceive a Black supervisor as inferior and lacking competence. Consequently, the White supervisee struggles to respect the Black supervisor's authority, especially if wider team members also show a lack of respect to the Black supervisor. Furthermore, the White supervisee can have more power in the dyad from White colleagues they can access who have structural, political and indirect power, influencing the supervisory relationship (Schultz & Warfield, 2010). Indeed, a supervisory relationship does not prevent a White supervisee from demonstrating racial microaggressions – brief and regular verbal, behavioural or environmental indignities that communicate hostile, derogatory or negative insults toward black people (Sue et al., 2007). Microaggressions and perception of institutional racism can and do cause stress (Clark et al., 1999).

According to Post and DiTomaso (2018) institutional racism leads institutions to essentially work better for White people than for Black so personal hostility in the form of macro or microaggression is not necessarily needed, as White people gain from existing structures. Simply put, 'the ultimate White privilege is the privilege not to be racist and to still benefit from the existence of racial inequality' (Post & DiTomaso, 2018, 61).

The argument is not that White people do not face any barriers in the workplace, as they do. Rather, along with barriers faced by White people, Black people frequently face additional ones. As Black British are not a homogeneous group (McInnis, 2018), in addition to race, implicit cultural bias may vary depending upon prejudices about countries of recent origin. Regarding support, some Black British communities function better than others. Furthermore, some individuals lack relatives in the same country, depending upon migration patterns within their family and the number who stayed in their country of origin (stayed home).

The question is raised why institutional racism or a system of White supremacy are needed? Is the satirical future at the start of this chapter what is feared? Fear of a Black planet (Eddo-Lodge, 2017)? I argue futuristic fear of Black people doing to White people what was done to them is misplaced. Fuller (1972/2016) calls for justice to replace racism. Even in the fictional futuristic *Black Panther* film (2018) the highly progressive East African country of Wakanda used the best technology and healing to benefit both Black and White people. Although fictional, it was researched and abundant with genuine African cultural practices such as Ubuntu (Murithi, 2006) which promotes betterment for all. So such a trajectory among others is reasonable to forecast.

Potential solutions

Black people have the capacity for self-preservation in the harshest of conditions, as demonstrated by the survival of enslaved ancestors and the Windrush generation of the UK. Therefore, the time has come to curtail commentary on racism in the hope the oppressor will stop (Parham, 2002; Nobles, 2006). The belt and braces approach would be to combine this with optimal rather than sub-optimal values, thinking and functioning for transformation (Myers et al., 2018; Parham, 2002). African psychology situates one in the field of psychology in relation to and from Africa (Ratele, 2017, 274). It expands the understanding of the human experience to include notions of energy (within and between persons), vibration and how that may influence mood, thought and interaction, and considers that increased healing may come from changes in community connectedness (Grills et al., 2018). Such strategies are needed for the spiritual subsistence of those characterised by dominant Western society as 'the other', in order for Afrikans[10] to build interior empires of strength for the journey ahead in multiple settings. It is no longer about 'stop doing X' but 'let's repair and heal damage done to our Black ancestors and start doing Y'. This is not to say the needs of other oppressed, marginalised and disempowered groups are not important. Furthermore, many Black people also belong to other disempowered and oppressed groups. But just as the response 'All lives matter' is made when 'Black Lives matter' is mentioned – yes, all lives do matter, but at the moment we are talking about 'Black lives'.

Why is this important? When clinical situations create frustrations for Black therapists lacking appropriate cultural frames of reference, our next generation is at risk of being 'young, gifted, and Black [ethnic] with inappropriate professional training' (Parham et al., 2011). This is training which does not meet the needs of their client or have meaning. What is sought is a framework which does not validate by comparison to White normative standards but ethical standards amongst the best in Afrikan functioning in constant exchange with the contemporary world (Karenga, 2010). However, this is not a 'nine to five' pursuit as healers need to integrate African-centred principles to their own life (Parham et al., 2011). Indeed, African-centred psychology is about life affirming principles that bring order and harmony to the life of both client and healer as the healer cannot facilitate spiritual enlightenment and illumination without such a state being accessible to themselves. It calls for use of healing concepts, tools and thinking abundant within Black communities in the therapy room, such as reflecting on proverbs and Ananse stories[11] (Goddard et al., 2020), and traditional West African wisdom concepts such as Adinkra symbols as a tool for wellness (Adom et al., 2016; McInnis, in preparation).

As we enter a new decade, we call for communities accepting of African-centred therapy to have it available, with African-centred supervision and organisational principles for high vibration functioning for all. A manifesto is a call to action (Elkins, 2009; McFall, 1991), so a new clinical psychology manifesto is called for which liberates, similar to that proposed for educational psychology (Wright, 2017). African-centred cosmology, ideology, principles and practices which could be included are numerous and outside the scope of this chapter, but include:

- notions of life-sustaining African cultural rituals
- remembering and respecting ancestors
- spiritness
- self-knowledge including racial identity as a key to well-being
- pursuit of optimal rather than sub-optimal ways of being and functioning
- purpose
- values such as Nguzo Saba
- principles such as Ma'at and
- dimensions of African self-consciousness such as Divinity, Teachability, Perfectibility, Free Will, and Moral and Social Responsibility (Karenga, 2010; Grills et al., 2018; Parham et al., 2011)

Conclusions

The thrust of this chapter is that implicit bias against Black people and preference for White people is fundamental to understanding the impact of institutional racism. Multiple institutions, governments and countries with this viewpoint have become a global system of White supremacy (Fuller, 2016).

It is acknowledged not all White people permanently uphold the system of White supremacy, but in my experience those who do often out-weigh or out-power those who don't. Furthermore, they are sometimes joined by Black people who want to improve their position within the system of White supremacy rather than dismantle it. My article in 2002 focused upon defining and detecting racism. Amos Wilson (Wilson, 1993; 2014) defined racism as a system for determining whose children will be fed first and whose last. This article alludes to theoretical models for understanding, betterment and transformation to a higher self, particularly for Black people. This is regardless of strategies which may be against Black people whether intermittent, seasonal or in residence (Myers et al., 2018; Parham et al., 2011). This chapter in no way says other forms of oppression do not exist, it is just that they may be better explored elsewhere. In this chapter some of the tactics of the system of White supremacy have been exposed. This is not presented to create unnecessary fear but awareness, as to be prepared can be forewarned. Organisations such as the Association of Black Psychologists (ABPsi) have an international reach developing therapies and offering initiatives designed to rescue, reclaim and restore African character, consciousness and conduct to recalibrate the future human trajectory of Afrikans (Grills et al., 2018).

Do we want more people with Black faces in psychology who peddle a paradigm which inappropriately works from a deficit model when it comes to the psychology of Blacks (Parham et al., 2011)? Or do we want more people who can make a difference 'seed by seed', making the very institutions which deliver services for clients abundant with approaches to meet people where they are?

Acknowledgements

I would like to thank the following for reading drafts and providing comments pre publication. Dr Edwin Nichols (Industrial and Clinical Psychologist, Nichols Associates), Professor Benson G Cooke (Professor of Counseling and Psychology, University of the District of Columbia and ex-president Association of Black Psychologists, ABPsi), Professor Huberta Jackson-Lowman (Professor of Psychology, Florida A&M University and ex-president Association of Black Psychologists, ABPsi), Professor Anthony Reddie (Extraordinary Professor of Theological Ethics and Director of the Oxford Centre for Religion & Culture), Dr Rebecca Wright (Educational Psychologist), Delroy Constantine-Sims (Chartered Counselling Psychologist), and Dr Pat Frankish (Clinical Psychologist, Director of Frankish Training and ex-president of the British Psychological Society).

This chapter is dedicated to the ancestors including my late father Jeremiah Eric McInnis (1928–2017). A man who planted seeds to bear fruit and shade for others to benefit. May we continue the journey started by our ancestors even when the road is tough, because we have a great past and an even greater future.

Notes

1 Kemetic refers to ancient Egyptian philosophies, cultures, spiritual practices and ways of being practiced in North Africa by Black people. These greatly influenced ancient Greek philosophers who developed Western psychology (Akbar, 1994; James, 1976).
2 Woke is a contemporary term to mean alert to injustice in society, particularly racism (Merriam Webster Dictionary).
3 'Big brother' is a term for an oppressive all-powerful government or organisation monitoring and directing people's actions. This phrase is widely used in the book *1984* by George Orwell (Merriam Webster Dictionary).
4 Black means individuals of high skin pigmentation with ancestors originating in Africa. It is acknowledged there is variation of skin pigmentation in Black communities and some experiences of Black communities may be common to other oppressed marginalised or disempowered communities. Reference to White people means Caucasian. It is acknowledged there are a multitude of variations within both Black and White communities.
5 Maafa in Kiswahili is a great disaster, African holocaust, dehumanising circumstance (Ani, 1997a, 12; Ani, 1997b, 3).
6 It is acknowledged in Western cultures, White (Caucasian) English is often respected as superior to White Irish/Scottish or Welsh. Furthermore, that White British is then often perceived or treated as superior to White Eastern European (those recently migrating from Eastern Europe).
7 The Equality Act (2010) sets out nine characteristics for which individuals are to be protected against discrimination. These are race, age, disability, gender reassignment, religion or belief, sex, sexual orientation, marriage and civil partnership and pregnancy and maternity.
8 HOMMS (Historically, Oppressed, Marginalised, Minority-status, and/ or Stigmatised groups) is a term used by Harrell (2018).
9 According to the United Nations, the descendants of the victims of enslavement, people of African ancestry all over the world; are today among the poorest and most marginalised groups. For instance, they have limited access to quality education, health services, housing and social security and all too often experience discrimination in their access to justice, and face alarmingly high rates of police violence, together with racial profiling (International Decade for People of African Descent 2015–2024, 2019).
10 The spelling of Afrika with a 'k' instead of a 'c' reflects reclamation of an identity that is different from that which has been constructed through colonialism. It refers to people of African ancestry with high skin pigmentation (Wilson, 1993, 2014).
11 Ananse (also spelt Anansi) is a folktale character taking the form of a spider with the spirit of wisdom and all knowledge of stories. Ananse can take the role of trickster and is often found in West African, African American and Caribbean folklore.

References

Adetimole, F., Afuape, T., & Vara, R. (2005). The impact of racism on the experience of training on a clinical psychology course: Reflections from three Black trainees. *Clinical Psychology*, 48, May, 11–15.

Adom, D., Asante, E. A., & Kquofi, S. (2016). Adinkra: An epitome of Asante philosophy and history. *Research on Humanities and Social Sciences*, 6(14), 42–53.

Akala (2018). *Natives: Race and class in the ruins of empire*. London: Two Roads.

Akbar, N. (1994). *Light from ancient Africa*. Tallahassee, FL: Mind Productions.

Ani, M. (1997a). *Yurugu: An African-centered critique of European cultural thought and behavior*. Lawrenceville, NJ: Africa World Press.

Ani, M. (1997b). *Let the circle be unbroken: The implications of African spirituality in the diaspora*. New York: Nkonimfo Publications.

Archibong, U., & Darr, A. (2010). *The involvement of Black and minority ethnic staff in NHS disciplinary proceedings*. A report of research carried out by the Centre for Inclusion and Diversity, University of Bradford on behalf of NHS Employers and NHS Institute for Innovation and Improvement. Available from: www.nhsemployers.org/~/media/Employers/Documents/Site CollectionDocuments/Disciplinary%20Report%20Final%20with%20ISBN.pdf (Accessed 1 October 2019).

British Board of Film Classification (2018). *Black Panther*, archived from the original on 3 February 2018, retrieved 30 September 2019.

Bowlby, J. (1988). *A secure base. Clinical applications of attachment theory*. London: Routledge.

Boyd-Franklin, N. (1989). *Black families in therapy: A multisystems approach*. New York: Guilford Press.

Boyd-Franklin, N. (2006). *Black families in therapy: Understanding the African American experience*. New York: Guilford Press.

Clark, R., Anderson, N. B., Clark, V. R., & Williams, D. R. (1999). Racism as a stressor for African Americans. *American Psychologist*, *54*(10), 805–816.

Cleland, J., & Cashmore, E. (2013). Football fans' views of racism in British football. *International Review for the Sociology of Sport*, *51*(1), 27–43.

Coghill, Y., & Kline, R. (2017). *Improving through inclusion. Supporting staff networks for Black and minority ethnic staff in the NHS*. Available at: www.england.nhs.uk/wp-content/uploads/2017/08/inclusion-report-aug-2017.pdf (Accessed 30 September 2019).

Cooke, B. G. (2018). Creating a stereotype of a race as dangerous, unintelligent, and lazy: Examining consequences of cultural and psychological conditioning in America, In P. Hampton-Garland, B. G., Cooke, & L. Sechrest-Ehrhardt, *Socio-economic and education factors impacting American political systems: Emerging research and opportunities* (pp. 1–28). Hershey, PA: IGI Global Publications.

Craig, U. (2013). *Shifting your paradigm for optimum health and longevity: A model of health and healing for African Americans*. Albemarle, NC: Gye Nyame.

Csikszentmihalyi, M. (2002). *Flow. The classic work on how to achieve happiness*. London: Random House.

Daiches, A. (2010). Clinical psychology and diversity: Progress and continuing challenges: A commentary. *Psychology Learning and Teaching*, *9*(2), 28–29.

De Houwer, J. (2019). Implicit bias is behavior: A functional-cognitive perspective on implicit bias. *Perspectives on Psychological Science*, *14*(5), 835–840. https://doi.org/10.1177/1745691619855638

Dennis, M., & Aitken, G. (2012). Incorporating gender issues in clinical supervision. In I. Fleming & L. Steen (Eds.). *Supervision and clinical psychology: Theory, practice and perspectives* (2nd Ed., pp. 118–141). New York: Routledge

DiAngelo, R. (2011). White fragility. *International Journal of Critical Pedagogy*, *3*(3), 54–70.

DiTomaso, N. (2015). Racism and discrimination versus advantage and favoritism: Bias for versus bias against. *Research in Organizational Behavior, 35*, 57–77.

Eddo-Lodge, R. (2017). *Why I'm no longer talking to White people about race*. London: Bloomsbury.

Elkins, D. N. (2009). *Humanistic psychology: A clinical manifesto. A critique of clinical psychology and the need for progressive alternatives*. Denver, CO: University of Rockies Press.

Equality Act (2010). The National Archives. Retrieved 28 September 2019.

Fein, S. (2018). The arc of racial stereotyping, prejudice and discrimination: social psychological perspectives. In J. M. Hayter & G. R., Goethals (Eds.). *Reconstruction and the arc of racial (in)justice*. Cheltenham, UK: Edward Elgar Publishing.

Fernando, S. (2017). *Institutional racism in psychiatry and clinical psychology: Race matters in mental health* (Contemporary Black History). London: Palgrave Macmillan.

FitzGerald, C., & Hurst, S. (2017). Implicit bias in health care professionals: A systematic review. *BMC Medical Ethics, 18*, article number 19.

Fuller, N. (2016). *The united independent compensatory code/system/concept: A compensatory counter-racist code*. Revised/expanded ed. Washington, DE: Nfj Productions.

Gentleman, A. (2019). *The Windrush betrayal: Exposing the hostile environment*. London: Guardian Faber Publishing.

Goddard, L., Rowe, D. M., McInnis, E. M., & DeLoach, C. (2020). The role of proverbs in African-centered psychology. *Alternation, 27*(1). *African-centered psychology: Illuminating the human spirit – spirit(ness), Skh Djr, Moya*. https://doi.org/10.29086/2519-5476/2020/v27n1a12.

The Guardian (2019). Boris Johnson urged to apologise for 'derogatory and racist' letterboxes article, 4 September 2019. Available at: www.theguardian.com/politics/2019/sep/04/boris-johnson-urged-to-apologise-for-muslim-women-letterboxesarticle (Accessed 8 October 2019).

Guilaine, K. (2014). There is no racism in clinical psychology: Personal reflections from another Black trainee, Blog, 19 October. Available at: https://racereflections.co.uk/2014/10/19/there-is-no-racism-in-clinical-psychology-personal-reflections-from-another-Black-trainee/ (Accessed 30 September 2019).

Gutherie, R. V. (1998). *Even the rat was white: A historical view of psychology*. London: Allyn & Bacon.

Grills, C., Nobles, W. W., & Hill, C. (2018). African, Black, neither or both? Models and strategies developed and implemented by the Association of Black Psychologists. *Journal of Black Psychology, 44*(8), 791–826.

Halton, W. (2009). Some unconscious aspects of organisational life. Contributions from psychoanalysis. In A. Obholzer & V. Z. Roberts (Eds.). *The unconscious at work. Individual and organisational stress in the human services*. Chichester: Routledge.

Harrell, S. P. (2018). Soulfulness as an orientation to contemplative practice: Culture, liberation, and mindful awareness. *Journal of Contemplative Inquiry, 5*(1). Available at: https://journal.contemplativeinquiry.org/index.php/joci/article/view/170. (Accessed: 8 October 2019).

Heatherton, C., & Camp, J. T. (2016). *Policing the planet: Why the policing crisis led to Black Lives Matter*. New York: Verso.

International Decade for People of African Descent 2015–2024 (2019). Available at: www.un.org/en/events/africandescentdecade/pdf/African%20Descent%20Booklet_WEB_English.pdf. (Accessed 17 October 2019).

Jackson-Lowman, H. (Ed.) (2014). *Afrikan American women: Living at the crossroads of race, gender, class, and culture*. San Diego, CA: Cognella Academic Publishing.

James, G. G. M. (1976). *Stolen Legacy*. San Francisco, CA: Julian Richardson Assoc.

Karenga, M. (2010). *Introduction to Black Studies*. 4th ed. Los Angeles, CA: University of Sankore Press.

Keyes, C. L. M. (2009). The Black-White paradox in health: Flourishing in the face of social inequality and discrimination. *Journal of Personality*, 77(6), 1677–1706.

Kick It Out (2019). Equality charter. London: The FA. Available at:www.thefa.com/competitions/the-fa-peoples-cup/kick-it-out (Accessed 10 October 2019).

Lintern, S. (2017). Exclusive: NHS England BME staff report widespread bullying. *HSJ*, 20 December. Available at: www.hsj.co.uk/workforce/exclusive-nhs-england-bme-staff-report-widespread-bullying/7021315.article (Accessed 29 September 2019).

MacPherson, W. (1999). *The Stephen Lawrence Inquiry*. Report of an Inquiry. [online] London: The Stationery Office. Available at: http://webarchive.nationalarchives.gov.uk/20130814142233/; http://www.archive.official-documents.co.uk/document/cm42/4262/4262.htm (Accessed 1 Oct. 2019).

The Mail Online (2011). We will use water cannons on them: At last Cameron orders police to come down hard on the looters (some aged as young as NINE), 11 August 2011. Available at: www.dailymail.co.uk/news/article-2024203/UK-RIOTS-2011-David-Cameron-orders-police-come-hard-looters.html (Accessed 29 September 2019).

McFall, R. M. (1991). Manifesto for a science of clinical psychology. *The Clinical Psychologist*, 44(6), 75–88.

McInnis, E. M. (2018). Understanding African beingness and becoming. *Therapy Today*, October, 28–31.

McInnis, E. M., & Moukam, R. R (2013). Black psychology for Britain today? *Journal of Black Psychology*, *39*(3), 311–315. DOI:10.1177/0095798413480663

McInnis, E. M. (2002). Institutional racism in the NHS and clinical psychology? Taking note of McPherson. *Journal of Critical Psychology, Counselling and Psychotherapy*, 2(3), 164–170.

McInnis, E. M. (in preparation). *Development of "Know Thy Self": Adinkra cards as a tool for self-illumination from an African centred perspective*.

McIntosh, P. (2003). White privilege: Unpacking the invisible knapsack. In S. Plous (Ed.). *Understanding prejudice and discrimination* (pp. 191–196). New York: McGraw-Hill.

Moylan, D. (2009). The dangers of contagion. Projective identification processes in institutions. In A. Obholzer & V. Z. Roberts (Eds.). *The unconscious at work. Individual and organisational stress in the human services*. Chichester: Routledge.

Murithi, T, (2006). Practical peacemaking wisdom from Africa: Reflections on Ubuntu. *Journal of Pan African Studies*, *1*(4), 25–34.

Myers, L. J., Anderson, M., Lodge, T., Speight, S., & Queener, J. E. (2018). Optimal theory's contributions to understanding and surmounting global challenges to humanity. *Journal of Black Psychology, 44*(8), 747–771.

Nobles, W. W. (2006). *Seeking the Sakhu. Foundational writings for an African psychology*. Chicago, IL: Third World Press.

Obholzer, A., & Roberts, V. Z. (2009). The troublesome individual and the troubled institution. In A. Obholzer & V. Z. Roberts (Eds.). *The unconscious at work. Individual and organisational stress in the human services*. Chichester: Routledge.

Odusanya, S. O. E. (2016). *The experience of qualified BME clinical psychologists: An interpretative phenomenological and repertory grid analysis*, vol. 1. Doctorate in Clinical Psychology thesis. University of Hertfordshire. Available at: https://pdfs.semanticscholar.org/bb09/3ecd9fed696792ba0d91a1b77bb243bf801c.pdf (Accessed 30 September 2019).

Orwell, G. (1949). *1984*. London: Secker & Warburg.

Parham, T. A. (Ed.) (2002). *Counselling persons of African descent: Raising the bar of practitioner competence*. New York: Sage.

Parham, T. A., Ajamu, A., & White, J. L. (2011). *The psychology of Blacks: Centering our perspectives in the African consciousness*. New York: Routledge.

Post, C., & DiTomaso, N. (2018). The effects of technical autonomy, gender, and family structure on innovativeness among scientists and engineers. In D. Embrick, S. Collins, and M. Dodson (Eds.). *Underneath the thin veneer: Critical diversity, multiculturalism, and inclusion in the workplace*. Leiden: Brill Academic Publications.

Ratele, K. (2017). Four (African) psychologies. *Theory and Psychology*, *27*(3), 313–327. Available at: https://doi.org/10.1177/0959354316684215

Reddie, A. G. (2019). *Theologizing Brexit: A Liberationist and Postcolonial Critique*. London: Routledge.

Reddie, A. G. (2003). *Nobodies to Somebodies: A Practical Theology for Education and Liberation*. Peterborough: Epworth Press.

Reeve, D. (2012). Psycho-emotional disablism in the lives of people experiencing mental distress. In J. Anderson, B. Sapey & H. Spandler (Eds.). *Distress or disability?* (pp. 24–29). Proceedings of a symposium held at Lancaster Disability, 15–16 November 2011, Lancaster: Centre for Disability Research, Lancaster University.

Schultz, M. S., & Warfield, J. (2010). *Transformative approach to improving the mental well-being of African American supervisors in cross-cultural supervision*. Association of Black Psychologists, 42nd International Convention, Chicago, IL, July.

Segundo, D. (2017). An exploration of the relationship between vicarious racism, police videos, and their impact on the Facebook consumer. Masters thesis, Smith College, Northampton, MA. https://scholarworks.smith.edu/theses/1919

Sue, D. W., Capodilupo, C. M., Torino, G. C., Bucceri, J. M., Holder, A. M. B., Nadal, K. L., & Esquilin, M. (2007). Racial microaggressions in everyday life: Implications for clinical practice. *American Psychologist, 62*(4), 271–286.

Turpin, G., & Coleman, G. (2010). Clinical psychology and diversity: Progress and continuing challenges. *Psychology Learning and Teaching*, *9*(2), 17–27. https://doi.org/10.2304/plat.2010.9.2.17

Vance, B. F. (2001). *From ghetto to community*. New York: Barnes & Noble.

Vara, R., & Patel, N. (2012). Working with interpreters in qualitative psychological research: Methodological and ethical issues. *Qualitative Research in Psychology*, *9*, 75–87. https://doi.org/10.1080/14780887.2012.630830

Vernon, P. (2019). The Windrush scandal was traumatic. Survivors need tailored mental health care. *The Guardian*, 9 October. Available at: www.theguardian.com/society/2019/oct/09/windrush-scandal-survivors-mental-health-care (Accessed 10 October 2019).

Washington Post (2018). Donald Trump is inspiring world leaders – just not the ones you'd think. He's turning mainstream conservatives across the globe into racists and nativists. 24 April. Available at: www.washingtonpost.com/news/made-by-history/

wp/2018/04/24/donald-trump-is-inspiring-world-leaders-just-not-the-ones-youd-think/ (Accessed 30 September 2019).

Wilson, A. (1993/2014), *The falsification of African consciousness: Eurocentric history, psychiatry and the politics of white supremacy.* New York: African World Infosystems.

Wood, N., & Patel, N. (2017). On addressing 'Whiteness' during clinical psychology training. *South African Journal of Psychology*, 47(3), 280–291. https://doi.org/10.1177/0081246317722099

Wright, R. (2017). *The stain of colonialism: Is educational psychology 'haunted' by the effects of colonialism? Using decolonised methodologies to interrogate practice.* DEdCPsy thesis, University of Sheffield. Available at: http://etheses.whiterose.ac.uk/20525/ (Accessed 17 October 2019).

Chapter 4

Re-embedding racism in psychology

Indigenising the curriculum in Australian psychology

Paul Duckett

Summary

In this chapter I discuss an important area of curriculum reform occurring in higher education called 'Indigenising the Curriculum' which aims to redress the under-representation of Indigenous people in the staff and student university population, and Indigenous knowledge in the university curriculum. This reform has been ongoing for around two decades and, though progress has been slow, there is some optimism that these reforms could create an anti-racism platform upon which we might build socially progressive programs of teaching in psychology. However, there is much to trouble such optimism in the discipline of psychology in Australia. Of concern is Australian psychology's impoverished understanding of its own history, uncritical adherence to a reconciliation framework and its paternalistic approach to Indigenous issues.

Overview and history of the Indigenising the Curriculum project

Indigenising the Curriculum (ItC) dates back to the 1990s. It centres on a recognition that colonisation has supplanted Indigenous knowledge systems with Eurocentric ones. Knowledge was stripped from the European colonies, loaded up with Western cultural assumptions designed to serve Western socio-economic and political interests and then returned to the colonies and used to reconfigure their social systems and institutions. In the early days this process was blatant, fervent and unapologetic, with the main cultural loading being Social Darwinism. Knowledge drawn initially from South America was taken to Britain, reconfigured to promote the Theory of Evolution and then exported back to the colonies in the form of Race Theory and Eugenics which was used to explain why Indigenous people were inferior to their European colonisers. By the 1960s a push back against this process took effect, largely due to the political activism of Indigenous people and a weakening of the Western political ability to maintain control over its colonies. This push back took time to impact teaching in higher education and when it did it took its most consolidated form through the ItC project. Work on ItC is being undertaken most notably in Australia, Canada, India, New Zealand, the United States and throughout the continents of Africa and South America. ItC is most often presented as the means to make the educational environment more accessible for Indigenous people, more respectful of Indigenous knowledge and to improve the retention of Indigenous students. Australia lags other countries, with the project only really taking hold around 2008 and progress has been slow since then.

History and present-day circumstance of Indigenous people in Australia

On 26 January 1788, the 'First Fleet' moored at Sydney Cove signalling the beginning of the British colonisation of Australia. At that time, the land was home to more than 230 Indigenous nations (Aboriginals and Torres Strait Islanders) who had held sovereignty over the land for more than 40,000 years. The British declared the land 'Terra Nullius' (land of no one) – a legal term signifying that the inhabitants of the land had no legal claim of sovereignty. This declaration was met with resistance by the Indigenous nations, resistance suppressed with military force by the British. An estimated Indigenous population of between 300,000 and 1 million prior to colonisation was reduced to around 60,000 in the years following colonisation. Despite that violence, the Indigenous nations did not cede sovereignty.

The state-sponsored genocide during the early years of colonisation was soon accompanied by control through social policies that enforced ghettoisation (Indigenous people were moved into missions and reserves), assimilation (Indigenous children were removed from their parents – the *Stolen Generation*) and welfarism (strict monitoring of social behaviours to ensure compliance with authorities). A broad level of institutionalised racism soon spread across the social, political and cultural domains through the embedding of paternalism and protectionism into white Australian culture. Today, paternalism and protectionism are the defining, seldom scrutinised, mainstream responses in Australia to Indigenous people – assumed by both the political left and right to be a morally appropriate response to the Indigenous 'problem'. An example of this protectionism was the Northern Intervention National Emergency Response Act of 2007 (known as 'The Intervention') which imposed upon Indigenous communities in Australia's Northern Territory health checks, alcohol bans and increased police surveillance. Though the Act was repealed in 2012, many of those measures remain in place in 2020 under the Stronger Futures in the Northern Territory Act. of 2012. The measures taken under these Acts have had little to no positive impact upon Indigenous people in the Northern Territory and their main effect has been to signal the government's willingness to infringe on the basic human rights of Indigenous people. Paternalism and protectionism are positioned against earlier forms of colonial violence so as to pass as benevolent forms of power, even though they are closely connected to that earlier form of violence. To be protected requires the protective intervention of the self-same forces that Indigenous people need protection from, and it maintains the identity of the protected as subjugated. The Catholic church had a particularly insidious role in violence undertaken in the name of protectionism, for which it eventually apologised in 1996.

The markers of the ongoing violence against Indigenous people can be found in the social and health statistics on Indigenous peoples that are now regularly reported under a Federally funded and administered 'Close the Gap' (CtG) strategy. That strategy was initiated in 2008 and its stated intention was to make improvements in Indigenous people's social and health outcomes by 2030. The inequalities it cited were shocking. Life expectancy for Indigenous people was on average ten years less for Indigenous people than non-Indigenous people, with 45% of Indigenous men and 34% of Indigenous women dying before the age of 45 (Australian Bureau of Statistics, 2009). The 12th annual CtG report published in 2020 reported that there had been no progress since 2008 to close the life expectancy gap and that there had been a widening gap regarding infant mortality (Australian Bureau of Statistics, 2016). The ineffectiveness of CtG is serving the interests of those who wish to promote the notion that the problems experienced by Indigenous nations are immutable and due to character defects of Indigenous people. In fact, the failures of the CtG strategy are attributable to the inherent paternalism of the approach adopted (driven top-down with insufficient consultation with Indigenous communities). Considering how the Australian government has given the CtG strategy woefully inadequate funding, how it is poorly planned and poorly coordinated, it along with 'Stronger Futures', resembles a protection racket.

Defining who is Indigenous

Any discussion of the history of Indigenous people in Australia traverses the politically contentious area of 'people naming'. It is an area replete with diverse definitions that operate between various politico-legal jurisdictions and heated, unreconciled debates. This has resulted in international definitions remaining generic and imprecise. The debates are heated largely because to be defined as Indigenous can afford a group specific rights over land and harvesting. Moreover, groups that engage in political activism are more likely to attract international public sympathy on the grounds of being an Indigenous rather than, say, an ethnic group (Sanders, 1989).

Colonisation and loss of sovereign powers sit at the heart of how the term 'Indigenous' is deployed internationally. Groups that claim Indigeneity but are largely denied that claim are those in positions of legal and political sovereign power. So, a colonised group primarily has a legitimised claim for Indigeneity if that group orients itself to the colonising group and accepts an identify defined by defeat and victimhood. The terms 'First People' and 'First Nations' are available and taken up by many groups as preferred, given they are not subjugating labels. Referring to First Nations in an Australian context has the effect of creating an identity that focuses on 40,000 years of lived culture rather than on 200 years of colonial occupation. But, the Indigenising the Curriculum project (ItC) cements the identity *Indigenous* into the debate. So, that is what I use in this chapter, but it should be read as a barbed term whenever it appears.

A brief history of psychology's racist practices against Indigenous Australians

Psychology has a shameful history in relation to Indigenous nations. It is not alone in that regard (see Connell, 2016). Psychology and anthropology made up a distinctly malicious partnership when they embraced theories linked to scientific racism during the early years of colonisation. This was tied to the popularity in academic circles from the late 1800s onwards of Social Darwinism which theorised that human development was on a trajectory that began with the simplistic and evolved to the complex. Indigenous people were characterised as less evolved humans and as childlike. For example, the Indigenous Protection Boards set up in the late 1800s to 'look after' the welfare of Indigenous people referred to their role as acting in *loco parentis*.

Some of the early work of psychology in Australia was motivated by a scientific concern that the Indigenous population of Australia was dying out and that there was a risk that their extinction would occur before science had properly gained sufficient knowledge about them (Chase & Turner, 1973). By the 1920s and 1930s that interest grew in intensity and scientists flocked to central Australia around the township of Alice Springs seeking out Indigenous communities. They congregated mostly on missions run by the Christian church and reserves set up by the government where they had a captive audience of Indigenous people to study.

Early psychometric testing of Indigenous people produced ambiguous results but was filtered to serve a particular agenda (Dudgeon et al., 2010). The research pushed to the public by politicians and the media was that Indigenous people performed poorly in key areas of psychological functioning (Kearney, 1966). This reflected an appetite of the politicians and non-Indigenous society for a narrative that explained the disadvantage experienced by Indigenous people and became a means for the States and Federal government of Australia to maintain resistance against Indigenous nations' political claims over land sovereignty.

That early psychological work proved rich pickings for political manipulation because it took little or no account of social, political and historical context. The trauma experienced by Indigenous people of being displaced from their homelands, the forced removal of children from their families and the deteriorating conditions on reserves in which they were placed that was causing death through starvation, largely did not figure in the psychologists' analysis. For example, during the early years of the Stolen Generation the prominent anthropologist-psychoanalyst Géza Róheim stated that the anxieties displayed by children who were forcibly removed from their parents were an expression of the Oedipal complex. The legacy of psychoanalytic work on Indigenous people in Australia remains today in the way that its focus on 'dreaming' has become a cultural trope for how Indigenous peoples' cultures are represented to non-Indigenous people. But Stanner, the anthropologist who coined the term 'The Dreaming', made a further important observation about Australian culture. He coined the phrase 'the Great Australian Silence' (Stanner, 1968) to sum up how Australians had effectively erased their memory of the violence of colonisation.

That forgetting was very evident in the work of psychologists along with their political naivety and insensitivity. No anticipation was made or responsibility taken for how knowledge produced by psychologists could be appropriated for harmful, political purposes or that there was any reason to cite or in any way acknowledge in their empirical reports the state-sponsored violence that was impacting the very population they were studying. Psychology appeared little troubled by this up until 2016 when it made a formal apology to Australian Indigenous people about its shameful past.

The APS, AIPA and the Australian Indigenous Psychology Education Project

In 2016, the Australian Psychological Society (APS) published its Apology on the APS website (APS, 2016). In its opening paragraph it acknowledged the poor social situation of Indigenous Australians and buffered this with a statement that it was important for psychologists to tell the stories of 'strength and resilience' of Indigenous peoples. The Apology listed some of the ways psychology had been complicit in the marginalisation of Indigenous people and then listed the APS's new commitments to Indigenous Australians. Those commitments are more or less what constitute the minimal standards for professional conduct specified in the APS Code of ethics published in 2007 (APS, 2007). The parsimonious nature of the APS commitments is troubling, but there is more that is troubling. The Apology's use of the term 'resilience' in no way pointed to how that concept might be understood from an Indigenous perspective – as an ecological, system-level, cosmologically centred concept (Kirmayer et al., 2011). Rather it was left to hang with no critical interrogation to alert the reader to take care with it and to not assume the Western understanding of it (i.e., that it is an individual trait). This is worrisome because the Western version of 'resilience' has become a marker for the solution offered by psychology for social ills – a focus on inverse, depoliticised risk factors. It depoliticises social problems by inviting the question: 'what can individuals do to protect themselves from social harm?' The Apology also refers to Indigenous peoples and communities and not to Indigenous nations, which side-lines Indigenous sovereignty issues (Riggs, 2013). And the de-politicisation of the harm being apologised for is further cemented in the final sentence of the Apology that cites the organisation's aspiration to improve Indigenous people's 'social and emotional wellbeing', with no mention of the need for political change. Indeed, the word political or any derivative of it is entirely absent from the document. There is much else to be troubled by in the Apology and I explore some more of that below, but first I consider what sparked the Apology and then what followed it.

The APS turn towards atonement was largely sparked in 1988 (Dudgeon et al., 2010) – the Bicentennial of the invasion of Australia by the British. It was a year charged with political debate over Indigenous sovereignty rights. 1988 was also the year that Australian psychology was seen to mature. It was the year it gained international recognition through hosting the 24th International Congress of Psychology. Despite it being hosted at a time of political heat where Indigenous issues were being discussed front and centre in Australian society, the only representation of Indigenous people at the congress was a section in a photographic exhibition called 'Indigenous Aspects of Australian Psychology' which consisted of a series of unapologetic photographs of Aboriginal skulls collected for scientific measurement. This was followed by an article published in the *Annual Review of Psychology* (Taft & Day, 1988) that offered a turgid portrayal of Indigenous people. For some members of the APS, this brought attention to the need for change. However, change was slow. At the 1991 Annual APS conference an APS interest group on Indigenous issues formed. In 1993 the APS established a working party whose remit was to produce guidelines for psychologists working with Indigenous people which much later became an adjunct to the APS Code of Ethics. But it wasn't until 2008 that the Australian Indigenous Psychologists Association (AIPA) formed in partnership with the APS and not until 2011 that the APS made a commitment to change through partnering with the AIPA to develop a Reconciliation Action Plan (RAP) (APS, 2012). Overall, the RAP was focused on working on areas of mutual interest and in bi-partnership with Indigenous people. There was no hint in the RAP of friction or potential conflict or any real sense that the project would capture any of the antagonism between Indigenous and non-Indigenous people that had characterised the politics of Australia for 200 years.

The developing role of the AIPA, the APS apology, and the RAP all led to the formation of the Australian Indigenous Psychology Education Project (AIPEP). The AIPEP was funded to develop frameworks, guidelines and strategies to introduce cultural responsiveness to the training of psychologists and to increase access to psychology training for Indigenous people. In 2016 the AIPEP published the *Curriculum Framework* document (AIPEP, 2016). In the 2019 Australian Psychology Accreditation Council (APAC) Accreditation Standards it is stated that APAC had become a co-signatory to a Statement of Commitment in relation to advancing the work of AIPEP and AIPEP frameworks. Thus, the AIPEP framework document became the first formalised attempt taken by psychology in Australia to Indigenise the Curriculum.

The framework document starts with promise, noting the sovereign claims of Indigenous people, but soon after turns towards a simplistic cultural analysis and away from a critical historico-political analysis, reflecting the tone of the APS Apology that preceded it. It takes on the tone of harmony and mutual interests, reflecting that of the APS RAP. But there are some interesting moments in the document, such as when it refers to historical injustices of colonisation and to racism in higher education. It holds some promise, particularly when it refers to the 'third space' approach advocated by Dudgeon and Fielder (2006). The 'third space' is that which sits between Indigenous and Western knowledge systems, or a space between the colonised and the coloniser. It is a space defined as full of friction, conflict and tension and is seen, for that reason, as the space that creates opportunities for a transformation of knowledge and new ways of knowing to emerge. But the overarching problem with the framework document is that the 'third space' appears an anomaly, as though it was something that leaked into the document but not something structurally integrated into it. Nowhere else in the document is there a recognition of the potential for disharmony and conflict. Nowhere else is there consideration that Indigenous and Western knowledge systems might sit fractiously together. But the slight muddying in the Framework document where there is some leakage that spoils such harmonic tones gives us an opportunity for teasing out factors that maintain psychology's political inertia regarding Indigenous issues.

How the indigenising project re-embeds a racist agenda into the Australian psychology curriculum

From reflecting on the APS apology, the APS RAP and the AIPEP Curriculum Framework document, we get a sense of Australian psychology's impoverished understanding of its own history, the problematic reconciliation framework it ascribes to, and the paternalist protectionism it exudes towards Indigenous people that embeds racist practices into the psychology curriculum.

History and forgetting

'The Great Australian Silence' is inscribed in psychology. The APS Apology and RAP somewhat acknowledge history but there is little sense that the scales are being rebalancing to fully account for the past. Psychology maintains a steadfast focus on engaging with procedural justice (that Indigenous people have access to decision-making processes) and restorative justice (making apologies and engaging in reconciliation processes) and much less on distributive justice (a shifting or resources from one group to another) or retributive justice (punishment based on *jus talionis*).

Institutionalised forgetting is something psychology has a habit of doing – providing a reconstructed historical account that serves its own purpose (Fryer, 2008). Harris (1980) described psychology as using history for ceremonial use (self-celebration) rather than for critical reflection. The latter disrupts the idea that psychology fits the mode of a fully fledged scientific profession. This might explain why scholarship in and critical teaching of the history of psychology has been in a precarious position within psychology (Chamberlain, 2010). A critical reading of the history of psychology reveals a sequence of internecine conflicts between various factions of the discipline. Rather than a linear progression of increasing canons of knowledge, we find circularity, contradiction and frequent self-inflicted implosions. We find a history pitted with a series of crises relating to its object of study, its method of analysis and whether psychology can be considered a 'proper' science. Further, a critical reading of its history reveals psychology is influenced heavily by political and cultural shifts in society to the point that it appears servile to economic and political interests rather than discovering empirically objective 'truths'. Particularly revealing is its attempts to supplant other disciplines, such as psychiatry, to gain power, prestige and resource – see, for example, the scandal reported in the 'Hoffman Report' (Hoffman et al., 2015). We find psychology keen to construct itself as a profession aligned to medicine and biology. As a political strategy this would make perfect sense given the ongoing insecure funding position of the humanities in higher education – particularly in recent years with increasingly right-leaning governments in the US, UK and Australia which has resulted in waning support for the arts, social sciences and humanities (Brock, 2014). So, psychology steadfastly promotes its links to biomedicine. Because of this and the lack of lessons learnt from the past, psychology continues to operate as a vessel to route and support eugenic ideas into Australian politics.

Reconciliation and remembrance

It might be argued that before non-Indigenous culture can begin to understand Indigenous culture, it needs to understand itself. The Australian historian Jim Berryman cites three key characteristics of Australian settler culture. These are: an acceptance of its British heritage; the adoption of a Judaeo-Christian belief system; and an adherence to the rational principles of enlightenment. Berryman states these three themes are particularly pronounced in Australian centre-right politics and among conservative commentators (Berryman, 2015). This context helps us pry out important points of disruption between Australian psychology and Indigenous knowledge systems that pivot around conflicting ontological and theological systems (see Sampson, 2000, for an important discussion of these). Australian psychology and more generally Western psychology stand on the primacy of the individual, the singularity of reality and a reductionist method of enquiry. This ontology aligns closely with the doctrine of the Catholic church (the most dominant religious institution in Australia), with the belief in *one God* translating through secular institutions into the ontology of *one Truth*. This is not a conspiratorial theory of the church smuggling God into psychology but more an appreciation of how religious doctrine becomes baked into a culture and those doctrines remain, even if only as a distant echo, in cultural and social institutions long after they have undergone a process of secularisation (Butterfield, 1961). The subtlety of the transmission of religious dogma through disciplinary practices such as psychology, are often latent and require deep interrogation, though they also are readily surfaced in such things as the APS member group Christianity and Psychology which aims to 'Increase the dialogue between Psychology and Christianity in mutually beneficial ways' (https://groups.psychology.org.au/capig/). What is certain is that psychology exists as a body of theory and practice with a complex body of inherited assumptions and ideas (Butterfield, 1961) and if these are not surfaced in the ItC project, the project will falter. Australian psychology, grounded in a monotheist, objectivist, reductionist scientific paradigm, conflicts starkly with Indigenous knowledge systems which are grounded in an animistic-polytheism, subjectivist, holistic paradigm. Under Indigenous knowledge systems to look for simple objective truths is not only culturally alien but deemed to be ultimately futile (Fatnowna & Pickett, 2002). This conflict extends to the very process undertaken by the APS, AIPA and AIPEP in relation to Indigenous people. The 'reconciliation' project starts with an assumption that the 'truth' will heal and rebuild a shattered past and that truth is one that is absolutist, objective and universal rather than contested, negotiated and transformative. You have to be certain about what you are sorry for before you can say you are sorry. This sits at the very heart of the reconciliation project that is structuring how Australian psychology is embarking upon ItC. Historical truths must be constructed into a singular account that is anointed with 'objective truth' and then any wrongdoings named in that account are cleansed through the act of confession. The theological undertones here are clear – confession cleansing the soul. It also renders Indigenous history through a Western lens, reinforcing the subjugated, powerless identity and victimhood of Indigenous people, the omnipotence of the all-conquering non-Indigenous people, and reinscribing the trauma of the former through the act of redemption and remembrance for the latter. In this way, saying sorry hurts more than it 'heals'. We must consider the echoes of Christian dogma in the ItC project in psychology and ask if the project is one more instance of colonial brutishness towards Indigenous people.

Infantilisation and paternalism

Indigenous people in Australia were treated, in the early days, as primitive and childlike. Little acknowledgement was given to the complex social and cultural systems that characterised Indigenous nations. The risk of ongoing infantilisation and paternalism is great, particularly for the ItC project in Australian psychology. With the apparent belief carried by that project that psychology's relationship with Indigenous knowledge systems and Indigenous nations will be harmonious we see a particular type of space being prepared for Indigenous knowledge to sit in the psychology curriculum. It is a space that reeks of what Probyn-Rapsey has referred to as 'the biopolitical power of paternalism and its accompanying rhetoric of "protection"' (Probyn-Rapsey,

2007, 92). Biopolitical power is that which aims to maintain life in a particular form (Foucault, 1976) – in this case, the maintenance of Indigenous people's subjugated position and the social regulation of their behaviour so as to cause no disturbance to the non-Indigenous population or their system of knowledge. The intent to create a harmonious space for Indigenous knowledge in the curriculum is not just pollyannaish, it is deeply paternalistic and infantilising. Indigenous knowledge is constructed as having some form of pristine, virgin purity that needs no discussion and no critical interjection, requiring no working on or working through but rather needs preserving – echoing the mission of the first psychologists to study Indigenous people in Australia before they became extinct. Little or no acknowledgement is given to the bleed between Indigenous and Western knowledge systems – mostly bled by the latter into the former (Coates, 2004) – and ruptures in Indigenous knowledge systems as attempts were made to phase them out of existence. This is despite it being known that Indigenous nations have been subject to more than 200 years of coercive assimilationist practices. I remember my first few visits to academic psychology conferences in Australia where I experienced the sharp sting of disapproval from the white Australian conference audience when I asked a critical question of an Indigenous speaker. The social norm was that you did not engage in scholarly debate with Indigenous speakers – they were there to be celebrated not critiqued. These processes romanticise Indigenous people and their knowledge systems as unadulterated and somehow otherworldly. This sets up Indigenous people and their knowledge systems, to paraphrase Povinelli et al. (1999), as failures of the very identity that defines them. Indigenous knowledge systems are not pure, pristine and certainly not without flaws. ItC is signalling to society that Indigenous knowledge is not to be taken seriously as competing knowledge systems but rather treated as unadulterated archaeological artefacts to be exhibited.

This problem of paternalistic protectionism is ratcheted up the moment Indigenous knowledge is brought into higher education, as universities are social institutions that reconstruct adults into children for the purpose of ensuring they are properly and fully socialised into the professional classes of society. The English common law notion of *loco parentis* was not only adopted by Indigenous Protection Boards in the late 1800s but also by universities. Though challenged during the 1960s and largely now no longer formerly operationalised in the university sector, its legacy endures in the administration of student loans and the organisation of student pastoral care. It can also be readily observed in the chatter among academics who still refer to their students as 'kids'. *Loco parentis* has also become resurgent recently through the guise of student satisfaction and student experience surveys that 'has highlighted the shift within institutions' priorities away from academic matters towards a concern with the personal, moral and social lives of students' (Hayes, 2015) and in the increased use of the term pedagogy to describe university learning and teaching philosophies – pedagogy meaning the teaching of children. We are already seeing the ItC project in Australia discussing 'Indigenous Pedagogies'. There can be no better institution than a university to continue the paternalistic, protectionist practices towards Indigenous people.

Can Australian psychology undertake a radical anti-racist stance through Indigenising the Curriculum?

For the ItC project in Australian psychology more work is needed to challenge the infantilising and patronising processes that sit both inside and outside of the higher education system, and psychology needs to re-examine the hegemonic position that reconciliation now holds over its work in this area. That position pushes restorative and procedural justice to the foreground and takes attention away from distributive and retributive systems of justice that not only are apposite but also form central parts of Indigenous moral systems. We need a more critically reflexive examination of the assumptions being carried into the ItC project and a more open discussion of the origin of those assumptions, including a clear and critical engagement with the history of Australian colonisation and the history of Australian psychology. To date, the ItC in Australian psychology feels very much at a nascent stage, which gives some optimism regarding possibilities to steer the project on a different course but disappointment regarding it taking this long to get to this point.

The latest documentation to come out of psychology in Australia, the AIPEP Curriculum Framework, does contain the seeds for a disruption but these need to be pushed to the surface. This could be achieved through the application of Critical Race Theory (see McLaughlin & Whatman, 2011; Milner, 2008) which is being used to important effect in South Africa to address the complex issues around colonised knowledge systems and reforming higher education (Carolissen et al., 2010, cited in McLaughlin & Whatman, 2011). Psychology might also be well served by increasing its connection to scholars working in the fields of critical geography and critical geopolitics (e.g. Wilcock and Brierley, 2012). The greater engagement with critical theory or, at the very least, critical reflexivity would ask psychology to consider how non-Indigenous Australians (particularly white Australians) have a subjective investment and material interest in depicting Indigenous people in certain ways and how Australian psychologists and higher education professionals share many of those same investments and interests and have codified them into their professional practices.

Nakata (2004) has argued that Indigenising the Curriculum is a project that is much more complex and contested than might appear from what we read in guideline documents that are coming out from various professions such as psychology. Nakata warns that any approach to the project that aims to simply put Indigenous knowledge 'in the mix' runs the serious risk of becoming a project of assimilation (Hauser et al., 2009). It can quickly become an extension of the colonialist project as Indigenous knowledges are deposited into higher education repositories ripe for trawling by transnational corporations – such as has happened to Indigenous health remedies that have been trawled by pharmaceutical companies and turned into corporate profit (Connell, 2016).

The reconciliation agenda cannot be given an uncritical passage. It needs to be considered whether Australian psychology's redemptive approach to Indigenous issues might be dovetailing into the centre-right political space in Australian culture and providing a point of least friction between Australia's conservative commentators and human rights activists. If it is, this is a dangerous compromised position to be adopting. It creates potent blind spots when the underlying ontological, theological and political positions are concealed. We have learnt as much from critical interrogation of the 'Truth and Reconciliation Commission' in South Africa (see Krog, 2000). One might say that psychology has replaced the notion of *terra nullius* with the notion of *spiritus nullius* (a denial that there existed or exists a theist grounding to the mainstream activities of the profession of psychology or in the ambitions of ItC, and a denial of the deep-rooted theological disruptions ahead).

Though the ItC project in Australian psychology is at an early stage, there is much more room for pessimism than there should be. Primarily this is in relation to the social institution where the project is being implemented – higher education. With a corporatist/managerialist turn taken by the higher education sector in Australia we are seeing increased pressure for academics to use institutional templates to structure their learning activities; external benchmarking of courses and programs; growth of an auditing culture to such dominance that almost every aspect of the learning and teaching environment is subject to panopticon systems of surveillance and control; crude, popularist ranking systems to increase competition between and within universities; and alignment of all teaching and learning practices and initiatives to corporate strategic plans. All of this is having the effect of narrowing the curriculum not widening it (Connell, 2016), the opposite direction required for the ItC project to succeed. The likelihood is that ItC will introduce Indigenous knowledge through quarantined and regulated spaces. This must be avoided so as to open the possibility of friction, antagonism, and ruptures such that Indigenous knowledge does not become wrapped in paternalism, delivered into the curriculum pre-sanitised and used to service the ideological interests of non-Indigenous groups (Milner, 2008). If ItC is done right, we should anticipate strong resistance from academics, administrators and managers within higher education as positions of privilege and power and systems of vested interest will be unearthed and this will cause concern and upset (Howlett et al., 2013). Paternalistic practices might be particularly difficult to shift given they are often sealed in the rhetoric of benevolence and philanthropy. The ItC project demands profound transformations if it is to disentangle itself from its racist past. Presently, Indigenous knowledge in the Australian psychology curriculum is given a space to be seen but not heard.

References

Australian Bureau of Statistics (2009). Experimental life tables for Aboriginal and Torres Strait Islander Australians, 2005–2007 *(Statement No.*3302.0.55.003). Available from www.abs.gov.au/ausstats/

Australian Bureau of Statistics (2016). Deaths, Australia (*Statement No.*3302.0). Available from: www.abs.gov.au/ausstats/

Australian Psychological Society (2007). *Code of ethics*. Melbourne: APS.

Australian Psychological Society (2012). *Reconciliation action plan*. Available from: www.psychology.org.au/reconciliation/

Australian Psychological Society (2016). *The APS apology to Aboriginal and Torres Strait Islander people*. Available at: www.psychology.org.au/About-Us/who-we-are/reconciliation-and-the-APS/APS-apology

Berryman, J. (2015). Civilisation: A concept and its uses in Australian public discourse. *Australian Journal of Politics and History, 61*(4), 591–605.

Brock, A. C. (2014). History of psychology. In T. Teo (Ed.), *Encyclopedia of critical psychology* (pp. 872–878). New York: Springer.

Butterfield, H. (1961). Reflections on religion and modern individualism. *Journal of the History of Ideas*, *22*(1), 33–46.

Chamberlain, J. (2010). Don't know much about history. *Monitor on Psychology*, 41(2), Available at: www.apa.org/monitor/2010/02/history

Chase, A., & von Sturmer J. (1973). 'Mental man' and social evolutionary theory. In G. E. Kearney, P. R. de Lacey, & G. R. Davidson (Eds.). *The psychology of Aboriginal Australians*. Sydney: Wiley.

Coates, K. S. (2004). *A global history of Indigenous people: Struggle and survival*. New York: Palgrave.

Connell, R. (2016). *Decolonising knowledge, democratising curriculum*. Available from www.uj.ac.za/faculties/humanities/sociology/.

Dudgeon, P., & Fielder, J. (2006). Third spaces within tertiary places: Indigenous Australian Studies. *Journal of Community and Applied Social Psychology*, *16*(5), 396–409.

Dudgeon, P., Rickwood, D., Garvey, D., & Gridley, H. (2010). A history of Indigenous psychology. In N. Purdie, P. Dudgeon, & R. Walker (Eds.). *Working together: Aboriginal and Torres Strait Islander mental health and wellbeing principles and* practices. Canberra: Australian Government Department of Health and Ageing.

Fatnowna, S., & Pickett, H. (2002). The place of indigenous knowledge systems in the post-postmodern integrative paradigm shift. In C. Odora Hoppers (Ed.). *Indigenous knowledge and the integration of knowledge systems: Towards a philosophy of articulation* (pp. 257–285). Claremont: New Africa Books.

Foucault, M. (1976). *The history of sexuality*, vol. 1. *An introduction*. New York: Random House.

Fryer, D. (2008). Some questions about "The history of community psychology". *Journal of Community Psychology*, *36*(5), 572–586.

Harris, B. (1980). Ceremonial versus critical history of psychology. *American Psychologist*, *35*(2), 218–219.

Hauser, V., Howlett, C., & Matthews, C. (2009). The place of Indigenous knowledge in tertiary education: A case study of Canadian practices in indigenising the curriculum. *Australian Journal of Indigenous Education*, 38(Supplement), 46–57.

Hays, D. (2015). As they compete to lay on the best student experience, universities mustn't forget the academic one too. *The Conversation*, 28 July. Available from https://theconversation.com/as-they-compete-to-lay-on-the-best-student-experience-universities-mustnt-forget-the-academic-one-too-45197.

Hoffman, D. H., Carter, D. J., Lopez, C. R.V., Benzmiller, H. L., Guo, A. X., Latifi, S. Y., & Craig, D. C. (2015). *Report to the Special Committee of the Board of Directors of the American Psychological Association: Independent review relating to APA Ethics Guidelines, national security interrogations, and torture (revised).* Chicago, IL: Sidley Austin LLP. Available from www.apa.org/independent-review/revised-report.pdf

Howlett, C., Ferreira, J., Seini, M., & Matthews, C. (2013). Indigenising the Griffith School of Environment curriculum: Where to from here? *Australian Journal of Indigenous Education, 42*(1), 68–74.

Kearney, G. E. (1966). *Some aspects of the general cognitive ability of various groups of Aboriginal Australians as assessed by the Queensland Test.* Queensland: University of Queensland, Department of Psychology.

Kirmayer, L. J., Dandeneau, S., Marshall, E., Phillips, M. K., & Williamson, K. J. (2011). Rethinking resilience from indigenous perspectives. *Canadian Journal of Psychiatry, 56*(2), 84–91.

Krog, A. (2000). *Country of my skull.* New York: Random House.

McLaughlin, J. M., & Whatman, S. L. (2011). The potential of critical race theory in decolonizing university curricula. *Asia Pacific Journal of Education, 31*(4), 365–377.

Milner, R. (2008). Critical race theory and interest convergence as analytical tools in teacher education policies and practices. *Journal of Teacher Education, 59*, 332–345.

Nakata, M. (2004). *Indigenous Australian studies and higher education (Wentworth Lecture).* Canberra: Australian Institute of Aboriginal and Torres Strait Islander Studies. Available from https://aiatsis.gov.au/sites/default/files/docs/presentations/2004-wentworth-nakata-indigenous-australian-studies-higher-education.pdf

Povinelli, D. J., Landry, A. M., Theall, L. A.., Clark, B. R., & Castille, C. M. (1999). Development of young children's understanding that the recent past is causally bound to the present. *Developmental Psychology, 35*(6), 1426–1439.

Probyn-Rapsey, F. (2007). Paternalism and complicity: Or how not to atone for the 'Sins of the Father'. *Australian Literary Studies, 23*(1), 92–103.

Riggs, D. W. (2013). Critical psychology in a context of ongoing acts of colonisation. *Annual Review of Critical Psychology, 10*, 79–87.

Sampson, E. E. (2000). Reinterpreting individualism and collectivism: Their religious roots and monologic versus dialogic person–other relationship. *American Psychologist, 55*(12), 1425–1432.

Sanders, D. (1989). The United Nations Working Group on Indigenous Populations, *Human Rights Quarterly, 11*(1989), 406–433.

Stanner, W. E .H. (1968). *After the dreaming. Boyer Lecture Series.* Sydney: Australian Broadcasting Commission.

Taft, R., & Day, R. H. (1988). Psychology in Australia. *Annual Review of Psychology, 39*(1), 375–400.

Wilcock, D. A., & Brierley, G. J. (2012). It's about time: Extending time-space discussion in geography through use of 'ethnogeomorphology' as an education and communication tool. *Journal of Sustainability Education, 3*, 1–28.

Chapter 5

'Something less terrible than the truth'

Oliver Twist and anti-semitism

Jonathan Calder

Summary

In this chapter the author examines the evidence for anti-semitism in the work of Dickens concentrating on book and film versions of the novel *Oliver Twist*. The chapter also highlights the history of boy martyrs and the concept of 'blood libel' well known to some Victorian readers of Dickens's work.

My great aunt's second husband was a joiner and, like many working men of his generation who aimed at self-improvement, he owned a complete set of Dickens. At young age – I would guess I was no older than 10 – I saw *Oliver!* at the cinema or possibly David Lean's film *Oliver Twist* on television, and decided that I wanted to read the original book. It was from Uncle Fred's set that I borrowed it.

I found *Oliver Twist* a dark and difficult book. The difficulty was inevitable given my age, but I was not wrong about the darkness. If we now think of it as a staple of Sunday afternoon television and full of benevolent bachelors and well-behaved orphans, we are wrong. It is a book about crime, injustice and the corruption of youth.

So I don't laugh at the Labour MP Victor Yates who asked in 1962:

> Does not the Minister agree that, even as recently as a week last Sunday, the broadcasting of a most brutal and bestial murder in the 'Oliver Twist' series at five o'clock – the peak hour – can have had nothing but a damaging influence, and was it not an exaggeration of Dickens? Will he use his powers to try to prevent this sort of thing?
>
> (Hansard, 1962)

But I do suspect that what was screened was not an exaggeration of Dickens at all and certainly not of the readings of the scene that Dickens performed later in life. In any case, Peter Vaughan must have made a great Bill Sikes.

As it turned out, there was an element of premonition about my early discovery of *Oliver Twist*. My own father walked out when I was 11, condemning me, if not to the workhouse, then certainly to the blacking factory for a while. This experience, on top of my reading of the novel, left me with a profound scepticism – perhaps too profound – about the systems set up to help the poor. So I was not surprised when I came across Foucault in later life: I had instinctively grasped his approach from my early encounter with Dickens.

Oliver Twist feels in many ways the novel that most justifies G. K. Chesterton's observation of Dickens' characters:

> It seems almost as if these grisly figures … were keeping something back from the author as well as from the reader. When the book closes we do not know their real secret. They soothed the optimistic Dickens with something less terrible than the truth.

There is, however, an element in the novel that I have never come to terms with, and that is the novel's anti-semitism.

In David Lean's classic film version of *Oliver Twist* Alec Guinness' portrayal of Fagin had been controversial, leading to riots when the film was shown in Germany and to trouble with the Hollywood censors. But, in an article now almost 30 years old (Calder, 1993) I treated this, alongside Victor Yates, as proof that the book was not the gentle read some had come to regard it as.

I was also pleased to find examples of British films of the 1940s being too controversial for Hollywood. I treated Guinness' Fagin as the equivalent of Dora Bryan's tart with a heart of gold in *The Fallen Idol* and the little naked goatherd in *A Matter of Life and Death*, both of whom alarmed the US censors of the day.

Yet today it seems incomprehensible to me that it was thought acceptable to put on screen a Fagin made to look like a figure from Nazi anti-semitic propaganda and that only three years after the world had discovered the enormity of the Holocaust – see Drazin (2013) for a discussion of the contemporary controversy. Yet the film is hardly alone in taking this attitude: think how Enid Blyton's children's books in these immediate post-war years continued to use Gypsies as stock villains.

Having acknowledged how problematic this anti-semitic stereotype is in David Lean's film, I can no longer ignore it when I return to the novel. And extremely problematic it is. An article in the *Independent* (Vallely, 2005) once quoted Milton Kerker, writing for the Jewish Theological Seminary of America:

> Fagin is no ordinary villain. He is the traditional medieval Jewish bogeyman, the Jew who is not a mere vicarious atavism of Satan, but the grotesque Jew, the crafty Jew in whose heart Satan is actually lodged.

And as the *Independent* journalist Paul Vallely (2005) went on to point out, Dickens introduces his villain with him standing before a fire, fork in hand, with a villainous and repulsive face, and matted red hair, which was just the hair traditionally worn by the devil in medieval mystery plays. Dickens, he reminds us, several times refers to Fagin as the 'merry old gentleman', an ancient euphemism for the devil, as is the phrase Bill Sikes uses when he says Fagin looks as if he has come straight from 'the old 'un without any father at all betwixt you' (Dickens, 1837–9/1985, 398).

The novel's antipathy to Fagin as a Jew is so deep that he is referred to as 'the Jew' more than 250 times in its first 38 chapters. In chapter 9 he is referred to as a Jew 29 times, but by his name only three. Such is the diabolical picture we are given of Fagin that we take it for granted he should be executed at the end of the novel. Yet, as John Sutherland (1997) has argued, it is not at all clear what capital offence he has committed. As Fagin himself asks when Oliver visits him in the condemned cell: 'What right have they to butcher me?' (Dickens, 1837–9/1985, 472).

The traditional defence of Dickens' depiction of Fagin is to indulge it as a youthful indiscretion, much as cabinet ministers are allowed to laugh off their drug offences at university when they are exposed by the press.

Key to this defence is the novelist's relationship with Eliza Davis, whose husband purchased his London home in 1860. Making an appeal for a donation to a Jewish charity, she wrote to Dickens:

> It has been said that Charles Dickens, the large hearted, whose works plead so eloquently and so nobly for the oppressed of his country, and who may justly claim credit [for], as the fruits of his labour, the many changes for the amelioration of the condition [of the] poor now at work, has encouraged a vile prejudice against the despised Hebrew.
>
> (Bloom, 2016)

And later in their correspondence she said: 'I hazard the opinion that it would well repay an author to examine more closely into the manners and character of the British Jews and to represent them as they really are' (Slater, 2011, 516–17). Dickens' response was twofold. He halted the reprinting of *Oliver Twist*, which was then halfway done, and edited the chapters that had not yet been set. This is why editions published to this day call Fagin 'the Jew' 257 times in the first 38 chapters but rarely in the 179 references to him in the rest of the book (Moskovitz, 1997).

Dickens' defenders also point to his final completed novel, *Our Mutual Friend* and the character of Riah. As Vallely (2005) points out, his goodness is almost as complete as is Fagin's evil and he offers an eloquent indictment of anti-Jewish prejudice.

> Men say, 'This is a bad Greek, but there are good Greeks. This is a bad Turk, but there are good Turks.' Not so with the Jews … they take the worst of us as samples of the best; they take the lowest of us as presentations of the highest; and they say 'All Jews are alike'.
>
> (Dickens, 1865/1997, 707)

It does not do to be dismissive of Dickens' intellect. Though this may seem a belated attempted to create a 'good Jew' to balance the portrayal of Fagin, at least one critic has taken the figure of Riah extremely seriously. Mardock (2005) suggests 'Dickens' attitudes toward actual Jews reflect the typical complexity of liberal Victorians', and offers a reading of Riah that looks back, not to Fagin and *Oliver Twist*, but to Shylock and *The Merchant of Venice*. He argues that Dickens uses Riah as an 'anti-Shylock' and uses him to critique his own society's presentation of the stage Jew.

It is good to be reminded that Dickens was a far more subtle writer than many critics allowed for much of the 20th century, yet a problem with this defence is that *Oliver Twist* soon became established in British culture in a way *Our Mutual Friend* never has. Everyone knows that Oliver asked for more, and probably that Nancy was murdered, even if they have never opened the book. Creating Riah shut the stable door, but Fagin is running riot to this day.

In large part this is down to the popularity of *Oliver Twist* with the makers of films and television programmes. So much so that the story that is known to the public is a simplified version told by David Lean in 1948 and by Lionel Bart and Carol Reed 20 years later in *Oliver!* It dispenses with the whole Maylie clan and curtails the intrigue around Oliver's parentage – his sinister half-brother Monks is nowhere to be seen.

It is hard to be too severe on this decision. Lean's film of *Great Expectations* is inevitably an inferior version of Dickens meticulously plotted novel. The film ends with Pip returning to Satis House and ripping down the cobwebbed curtains so the light streams in, which is something that in the novel he once imagined as a young man, only to laugh at himself later for thinking such a trite resolution possible (Dickens, 1860–1/1985, 253).

Oliver Twist is not that sort of novel: it is remembered for the power of its characters and set pieces rather than for the elegance of its plotting. Reading it, you are aware that it was written in instalments and sense that much of the plot is set out towards the end of the book in an attempt to bring some kind of order to the extraordinary scenes Dickens created.

He is not wholly successful. For, as Morgentaler (2000) reminds us, Oliver's resemblance to his mother is so strong that it is evident to Mr Brownlow the first time he lays eyes on the boy even though he knows her features only from a portrait.

Yet the plot also requires Oliver to bear an equally striking likeness to his father. So Brownlow recalls towards the end of the novel:

> Even when I first saw him in all his dirt and misery, there was a lingering expression in his face that came upon me like a glimpse of some old friend flashing on one in a vivid dream.
>
> (Dickens, 1837–9/1985, 438)

Just as Fagin's appearance is enough to damn him and condemn him to the gallows, so Oliver's saves him and restores him to his rightful station.

The excision of Monks from the plot in these later tellings of the story has removed a deeper strain of anti-semitism from the novel. Monks is the older half-brother of Oliver and wishes to deprive the latter of the inheritance that their father settled upon the younger boy. No doubt there is another version of the story in which Monks is seen as being wronged by this arrangement, but there is at least a condition in the father's will that places an obstacle in the way of Oliver inheriting his fortune:

> If it were a girl, it was to inherit the money unconditionally; but if a boy, only on the stipulation that in his minority he should never have stained his name with any public act of dishonour, meanness, cowardice, or wrong. He did this, he said, to mark his confidence in the other, and his conviction – only strengthened by approaching death – that the child would share her gentle heart, and noble nature.
>
> (Dickens, 1837–9/1985, 458)

It is this clause that Monks seeks to exploit and his chosen instrument is Fagin.

As Nancy tells Rose Maylie during the meeting that seals her fate, because Sikes believes she has informed on him:

> A bargain was struck with Fagin, that if Oliver was got back he should have a certain sum; and he was to have more for making him a thief, which this Monks wanted for some purpose of his own.
>
> (Dickens, 1837–9/1985, 362–3)

We know better than Rose what Monks' purpose was.

Those murdering Jews

This dishonouring or defiling of an innocent Christian boy at the hands of a Jew is reminiscent of the 'blood libel', which accuses Jews of murdering Christian children so they can use their blood as part of religious rituals. Yet it feels more closely related to the local cults of boy martyrs that flourished in England in the 12th and 13th centuries.

The best known of these cults, dating from 1255, is that of Little St Hugh of Lincoln, whose shrine still stands in the cathedral and who is mentioned in Chaucer's *Prioress's Tale* and Marlowe's *The Jew of Malta*. Mundill (1998), however, suggests the first such cult is that of St William of Norwich, which dates from 1144, whose shrine was believed to the site of miracles.

Mundill identifies further examples of these cults at Gloucester in 1168, Bury St Edmunds in 1181, Bristol in 1183 and Winchester in 1892. He traces further cases of Jews being accused or convicted of the murder of a Christian child into the 13th century, including one where the supposed victim was found alive and another where the boy's mother was later charged with murder. In 1244 a shrine to a dead baby whose body supposedly bore the marks of ritual murder was erected at St Paul's Cathedral.

You can still find the remnants of the shrine to 'Little St Hugh' (he was never canonised by Rome) in Lincoln cathedral. It survived intact until the Reformation, or possibly even until Cromwell's Commonwealth, but a recent visitor (Backwatersman, 2012) found that:

> the bones of Hugh (who, of course, never asked for any of this) are relegated to an obscure aisle, accompanied by an apology which states (quite correctly) that 'such stories do not rebound to the credit of Christendom' and ends 'so let us pray: forgive what we have been, amend what we are, and direct what we shall be.'

According to Morrell (1993), the shrine was moved to its current location and the apology put in place in 1959. The apology replaced a straightforward telling of the story of Hugh's martyrdom because, in the words of the Dean, the Revd D. C. Dunlop, the Dean and Chapter did not wish 'to see things that are untrue up on the walls of the cathedral'.

That untrue thing was an anti-semitic fantasy, the full version of which was recorded by the 13th-century chronicler Matthew Paris (quoted in Hill, 1948, 224–5).

> This year about the feast of the apostles Peter and Paul, the Jews of Lincoln stole a boy called Hugh, who was about eight years old. After shutting him up in a secret chamber, where they fed him on milk and other childish food, they sent to almost all the cities of England in which there were Jews, and summoned some of their sect from each city to be present at a sacrifice to take place at Lincoln, in contumely and insult of Jesus Christ. For, as they said, they had a boy concealed for the purpose of being crucified; so a great number of them assembled at Lincoln, and then they appointed a Jew of Lincoln judge, to take the place of Pilate, by whose sentence, and with the concurrence of all, the boy was subjected to various tortures.

Paris goes on to detail the boy's tortures, which mirror Christ's suffering on the cross, in loving detail before concluding:

> And after tormenting him in diverse ways they crucified him, and pierced him to the heart with a spear. When the boy was dead, they took the body down from the cross, and for some reason disembowelled it; it is said for the purpose of their magic arts.

Goller (1987) tells us what happened once the boy's body was found:

> Hardly had the suspicion been voiced that the Jews of Lincoln had committed a ritual murder when Copin, the Jew in whose courtyard the body had been found, was imprisoned and threatened with torture and death, should he not tell the truth. With his statement we are already in the realm of fiction.

It is from Copin's statement that the idea that the whole Jewish community in England was implicated in the boy's death comes – the same 'admission' was forced from a Jew in Norwich in 1144. Henry III came to Lincoln to supervise the investigation himself and 18 Jews were hanged in London because they refused to testify in front of a purely Christian jury. A further 72 were later pardoned and released from the Tower of London.

Goller also traces how the legend of Little St Hugh developed through folk ballads and nursery rhymes. One telling of it, the bowdlerised folk song Sir Hugh, survives to this day and was recorded by Steeleye Span in 1975.

What shall we do with Oliver?

What, then, to do about *Oliver Twist*? One approach is that adopted by a Mr Rosenberg, who in 1949 called for both *Oliver Twist* and *The Merchant of Venice* to be dropped from the curriculum of schools in the city of New York because the tended to 'engender hatred of the Jew as a person and as a race'. The school board declined to do so, leading to a court case which Mr Rosenberg lost (American Library Association, 2017).

Though this chapter was written in those strange weeks when libraries were closed, a statue was thrown into Bristol harbour and the media was obsessed with the fate of many more, there has never been much appetite for such an outright ban on *Oliver Twist*; Dickens' place in the canon now feels more secure than it did 50 or 100 years ago.

And we can certainly change the literary classics. Each reading of a book is a new reading of it as the meaning of a text lies in the relation between it and its readers. It may be that it is precisely those novels that are unstable, that are most open to new readings as society changes around them, that remain alive to us.

The idea that reading and arguing about such novels has the potential to tell us something about the way we should live our lives now feels hopelessly old-fashioned, but it can still be defended. Richard Rorty (1989), an impeccably postmodern and radical philosopher whose work still gives off a whiff of brimstone to some in his own discipline, used discussions of Proust, Orwell and Nabokov to elucidate his ideas in when he wrote *Contingency, Irony, and Solidarity*.

Oliver Twist proved a particularly unstable text as it was retold from the start. Dickens was plagued by pirated editions of his early novels, some of which tried to fool the reader into thinking they were the real thing while others burlesqued the original.

That instability, as we have seen, carried over into the film adaptations as directors struggled with the novel's byzantine plot and has been equally apparent more recently as adaptations have looked for ways of challenging, curbing or disguising the novel's anti-semitic elements.

Lionel Bart chose the first route, giving Fagin all the best tunes. Though radio stations in the 1960s were obsessed with 'Food Glorious Food', it is the sinuous music of 'Reviewing the Situation' that the viewer is likely to remember. Add in the lyrics where Fagin declares 'I'm finding it hard to be really as black as they paint' and Dickens' devilish villain is taking the first steps on the path to becoming a hero – or at least an anti-hero.

In 1999 Alan Bleasdale wrote a television adaptation that, though it altered many details, took the novel's plot more seriously than Bart did in that we saw Oliver's father and Monks in the first episode, with Oliver not appearing until the second.

Talking to the *Guardian* (Brown, 1999), Bleasdale identified three problems with the novel: Dickens' love of implausible coincidence, his sentimentality and its anti-semitism. 'I did not want to portray a Jewish person or an immigrant in this day and age as an out-and-out villain', said Bleasdale, but he retained the speech rhythms of Dickens's original Fagin. So when Robert Lindsay, who was to play Fagin, read the script he said 'I can't play him as other than Jewish'. The portrayal, said Bleasdale, was softened by making Fagin 'a failed magician, an immigrant from Prague, who seduces the children through magic, hot sausages and gin', suggesting it owed much to the ghost of Ron Moody from *Oliver!*

The problem of Dickens' characterisation of Fagin became more acute in Roman Polanski's 2005 film adaptation of the novel, given the director's own family background. He was born in Paris in 1933 to Polish-Russian parents, and the family moved back to Kraków three years later. The city became the capital of German-occupied Poland in 1939 and a ghetto, where the Polanski family were confined along with its remaining Jews, was created there in 1941. A *Guardian* feature (Pulver, 2015) described Polanski as recalling seeing Jews executed in the street by the SS and his own escape from the ghetto in 1943 after his parents had been deported to concentration camps. His parents were both sent to the camps and his mother was to die in Auschwitz.

Polanski's Fagin was Ben Kingsley, who was quoted by *The Jewish News of Northern California* (Fox, 2005) discussing the novel's backstory when the film was released in the United States:

> I speculated that maybe his grandparents came to England with this little child who didn't speak a word of English. ... They were holed up in some strange place in the East End. [And] these Russian-speaking grandparents died when he was still a child. Then he was out in the streets fending for him-self and then you have two orphans in the same room. You have Fagin

> and Oliver, having a strange understanding of one another and a strange interdependence, and eventually a bond between them.

He told the newspaper:

> It was a very severely restricted society. The professional avenues were severely limited for what Ashkenazis could do in London. It basically came down to you can buy and sell second-hand clothes, you can be a rag-picker and you can unofficially lend money.
>
> So the legal openings for Fagin – for my young, abandoned Fagin – were severely limited. … In the East End, you learned to live off your wits as you would in Rio de Janeiro now. You become a street kid, and your aspiration would be to be the toughest kid on the street and then to have your own street kids when you grow up. It's a very, very limited perception of what the world is, which Fagin has.

He also said that he and Polanski had not discussed Fagin's Jewishness:

> Because of our great affection for one another, that debate never infected the workspace or worried us. … I was just allowed to explore Fagin as a collapsed patriarch, as a distorted parent figure. Terribly corrupted and distorted, but somewhere inside is that tradition – he mentions it when he's dressing [Oliver's] wound. 'Handed down from father to son, father to son,' and then he stops and says, 'But I don't know where from.' As if his tribal memory snapped. And I found that very sad in him.

Yet the scriptwriter Ronald Harwood, himself Jewish like Polanski, found it easy to do away with the novel's anti-semitism:

> If you read the book, only Dickens refers to him as a Jew,' says Harwood, who was born in South Africa and moved to England as a teenager in 1951. 'The characters never say, "Oh, Fagin, the dirty Jew" or "Fagin, the evil Jew." So as long as I'm only dramatizing the scenes, I can be faithful to that.'

It has been said that we only know Fagin is Jewish because Dickens tells us he is. There is no sign of religious observance in anything he says or does in the novel.

I quoted Ben Kingsley at such length because those words suggest he is familiar with the most radical retelling of *Oliver Twist*. This is to be found in the graphic novel *Fagin the Jew* by Will Eisner (2003 – also discussed in Kaufman, 2017). Eisner explains its genesis in his introduction:

> A few years ago, as I was examining folk tales and literary classics for possible graphic adaptation, I became aware of the origins of ethnic stereotypes we

> accept without question. Upon examining the illustrations of the original editions of *Oliver Twist*, I found an unquestionable example of visual defamation in classic literature. The memory of their awful use by the Nazis in World War II, one hundred years later, added evidence to the persistence of evil stereotyping. Combating it became an obsessive pursuit, and I realized that I had no choice but to undertake a truer portrait of Fagin by telling his life story in the only way I could.

Eisner's Fagin tells his story in the condemned cell, though as Sutherland (1997) points out, it is not at all clear from Dickens' novel that he has committed a capital crime – perhaps readers have always taken the devilishness that surrounded the character as justification enough.

Fagin's parents, he tells us, arrived in London from somewhere in Middle Europe – 'How they made the journey, God only knows' – and found a community where Jews were not subject to pogroms or special laws. They also found, though, that the Ashkenazim, Middle European Jews like themselves, were seen as socially inferior to the established Sephardim from Spain and Portugal.

In an afterword Eisner suggests that both Dickens and his illustrator George Cruikshank presented Fagin as a classic stereotypical Jew 'based on ill-considered evidence, imitation and popular ignorance'. The novel's pictures of Fagin, he argues, are based on the appearance of the Sephardim, whose features, hair and complexions were the result of 400 years living among Latin and Mediterranean peoples. Ashkenazi Jews, by contrast, had come to resemble the Germans among whom they lived, and there were many blond Jews 'as a result of rapes that occurred during pogroms'. The novel's reliance upon such old stereotypes confirms the theory that its anti-semitism has deep roots.

Eisner gives the young Fagin suitably Dickensian adventures. As a little boy he is put to work peddling needles and buttons on the London streets. When his father is murdered and his mother dies from illness and hunger, he is taken into the household of a wealthy Jewish man, Eleazer Salomon, who dreams of establishing a school for the Jewish boys of the East End. Fagin is 17 when the school is founded and he goes to work there as a caretaker, only to be thrown out when he falls in love with Rebecca Lopez, the daughter of another of its wealthy backers. With little to fall back on, Fagin turns to crime and is eventually caught and transported for handling stolen goods.

Returning to London after ten years of slavery he finds crime is still the only career open to him:

> Broken in body, in fragile health, I was in appearance a shuffling greybeard, the result of the horrors of penal life and imprisonment.
>
> However, I still had me wits about me. Sharper than ever were my skills, which were honed in the penal colonies.

> In London, I had finally established myself. I was no longer naïve: gone was the promise that fuelled my hope of a grand future. I was what the urchins who worked for me would one day become.

From then on Eisner tells the tale much as Dickens told it. There is, though, a final act of retelling which sees Fagin positioned as a wronged child every bit as much as Oliver. For Eleazer Salomon turns out to have been a benevolent bachelor like Mr Brownlow; he regarded the young Fagin as his son and was heartbroken when he disappeared after being thrown out of the school by Rebecca Lopez's father.

Unlike Oliver, Fagin was never rescued: rather than being his fortune, his face damned him. Salomon's money went to the Lopez family instead, to be inherited by Oliver Twist when he married Rebecca Lopez's daughter.

To follow the insight of G. K. Chesterton (another favourite writer whose anti-semitism I should have been more troubled by) we now know the truth that Dickens' characters were hiding from him in *Oliver Twist*. It is a truth at once terrible and tawdry.

References

American Library Association (2017). Notable First Amendment court cases. www.ala.org/advocacy/intfreedom/censorship/courtcases Accessed 8 July 2020.

Backwatersman (2012). Forgive what we have been, amend what we are. *The Crimson Rambler*. Retrieved from https://backwatersman.wordpress.com/2012/10/21/forgive-what-we-have-been-amend-what-we-are-little-saint-hugh-of-lincoln Accessed 8 July 2020.

Bloom, C. (2016). Charles Dickens' anti-Semitism: How a Jewish woman helped set him straight. *Jewish Currents*, Spring. Retrieved from https://jewishcurrents.org/charles-dickenss-anti-semitism/ Accessed 8 July 2020.

Brown, M. (1999). Oliver with a twist. *The Guardian*, 22 November. Retrieved from www.theguardian.com/media/1999/nov/22/pressandpublishing.classics Accessed 8 July 2020.

Calder, J. (1993). The persistence of Oliver Twist. *Changes: An International Journal of Psychology and Psychotherapy, 11*(4), 319–326.

Dickens, C. (1837–9/1985). *Oliver Twist*. Harmondsworth: Penguin.

Dickens, C. (1860–1/1985). *Great Expectations*. Harmondsworth: Penguin.

Dickens, C. (1865/1997). *Our Mutual Friend*. Harmondsworth: Penguin.

Drazin, C. (2013). Dickens's Jew – from evil to delightful. *Jewish Chronicle*, 3 May. www.thejc.com/comment/opinion/dickens-s-jew-from-evil-to-delightful-1.44612. Accessed 8 July 2020.

Eisner, W. (2003). *Fagin the Jew*. New York: Doubleday.

Fox, M. (2005). A twist in this Oliver: Ben Kingsleys wistful Fagin. *Jewish News of Northern Carolina*, 16 September. www.jweekly.com/2005/09/16/a-twist-in-this-oliver-ben-kingsley-s-wistful-fagin. Accessed 8 July 2020.

Göller, K. H. (1987). 'Sir Hugh of Lincoln': From history to nursery rhyme. In B. Engler & K. Müller (Eds.). *Jewish life and Jewish suffering as mirrored in English and American literature* (pp. 17–31). Paderborn: Schöningh.

Hansard. (27 March 1962) HC Deb 656, col 988. https://api.parliament.uk/historic-hansard/commons/1962/mar/27/television-programmes-scenes-of#column_988. Accessed 8 July 2020.

Hill, F. (1948). *Medieval Lincoln*. Cambridge: Cambridge University Press.

Kaufman, H. (2017). A new order: Reading through pasts in Will Eisner's neo-Victorian graphic novel, Fagin the Jew. In A. M. Jones & R. N. Mitchell (Eds.). *Drawing on the Victorians: The palimpsest of Victorian and neo-Victorian graphic texts.* Athens, OH: Ohio University Press.

Mardock, J. D. (2005). Of daughters and ducats: Our Mutual Friend and Dickens's anti-Shylock. *Borrowers and Lenders: The Journal of Shakespeare and Appropriation, 1,* 2. https://openjournals.libs.uga.edu/borrowers/article/view/2153/2044. Accessed 8 July 2020.

Morgentalter, G. (2000). *Dickens and heredity: When like begets like.* Basingstoke: Macmillan.

Morrell, R. W. (1993). The mystery of St Hugh's Well, Lincoln. *At the Edge.* www.indigogroup.co.uk/edge/Sthugh.htm. Accessed 8 July 2020.

Moskovitz, H. (1997). From Fagin to Riah: How Charles Dickens looked at the Jews. *The Charles Dickens Page.* www.charlesdickenspage.com/from-fagin-to-riah.html. Accessed 8 July 2020.

Mundill, R. R. (1998). England's Jewish solution: Experiment and expulsion, 1262–1290. *Cambridge Studies in Medieval Life and Thought*; 4th series, 37. New York: Cambridge University Press.

Pulver, A. (2015). Roman Polanski revisits Holocaust experiences in candid interview. *The Guardian,* 16 December. www.theguardian.com/film/2015/dec/16/roman-polanski-holocaust-experiences-candid-interview-video-testimony. Accessed 8 July 2020.

Rorty, R. (1989). *Contingency, irony, and solidarity.* Cambridge: Cambridge University Press.

Slater, M. (2011). *Charles Dickens.* New Haven, CT: Yale University Press.

Sutherland, J. (1997). *Can Jane Eyre be happy? More puzzles in classic fiction.* London: Allen & Unwin.

Vallely, P. (2005). Dickens' greatest villain: The faces of Fagin. *Independent,* 7 October. www.independent.co.uk/arts-entertainment/films/features/dickens-greatest-villain-the-faces-of-fagin-317786.html. Accessed 8 July 2020.

Chapter 6

Racism and the rights movement

Lauren Tenney

Summary

This chapter explores racism within and beyond the psychiatric survivor movement. It discusses some current issues faced by those who qualify to work in the US peer industry, in terms of the state-sponsored system's racist practices. Our movement must acknowledge and eliminate these racist and classist tendencies and support abolition of slavery in all of its forms, including as a form of punishment as allowed in the US by the Thirteenth Amendment, and how in prisons and jails, and in silent tandem in psychiatric institutions, slavery is maintained via the psy industries.

Introduction

I write this from the perspective of someone who was locked up in a psychiatric institution when I was 15 years old. I now live in a 48-year-old queer body and witchy soul that could be categorically described as having Italian Roman Catholic, Irish, Ashkenazi Jewish, and Eastern European roots.

I will never experience or understand from a first-hand knowledge the clear racist practices exhibited by psychiatry. I also will never experience, at the macro level, the racism exhibited in the environmental psychology of America. I am aware of the multiple privileges I experience. My original work in the psychiatric survivor movement was as a young person aging out of the Youth Rights Movement. My transformation from 'mental health consumer' to 'psychiatric survivor' was nearly immediate upon learning of the Mental Patients Liberation Movement in the 1990s. My goals became to strive for mutual support and combat psychiatric oppression and torture. I later more firmly began supporting the human rights movement for people with psychiatric histories and made analyses of how the Declaration of Human Rights is violated at multiple juncture points, including violations of the human rights to be free from torture, the condition of slavery or being murdered.

Psychiatric oppression includes being institutionalised against one's will and incarcerated for no crime committed. While incarcerated, psychiatric oppression creates the condition where one is to be subjected by direct experience, or as a witness without the power to act or intervene, the use of physical holds, mechanical restraints, chemical restraints and solitary confinement as forms of 'treatment' and social and behavioural control.

To be psychiatrically oppressed is to be subjugated as patient and have all claims of self-knowledge revoked and dismissed. It is to be isolated from friends and family without free communication – to be subjected to a host of psychiatric products and procedures, potentially including pills, electric shock and brain surgery. To be without the right to choose or enact informed consent in one's own supposed medical treatment is the condition of psychiatric oppression. It is to have your right to refuse medical treatment protected if you comply and revoked as soon as you no longer comply.

Judi Chamberlin (1990) also acknowledged the problem of expectation by the people in the field of psychiatry for the patient to exhibit compliance to their orders:

> Let's look at this word 'compliance.' My dictionary tells me it means 'acquiescent,' 'submissive,' 'yielding.' Emotionally healthy people are supposed to be strong and assertive. It's slaves and subjects who must be compliant. Yet compliance is often a high value in professionals' assessments of how well we are doing. Being a good patient becomes more important than getting well.
>
> (p. 51)

The rights movements, whatever they were called at varying periods of time, dating back to the 19th-century Lunatics Liberation Movement in New York State, have always had an end of state-sanctioned forced psychiatry as a goal. The use of force in psychiatry is not a new idea. As far back as the Managers Logs of the Utica State Lunatic Asylum, the message was that it was better to bring an inmate to the asylum by force, rather than deception (cf. Utica State Lunatic Asylum Managers Log, 1844; Asylum log, 2020).

In the 19th century, as now, there was absolutely no biological evidence for any supposed form of insanity to legitimise forced involvement with the mad doctors, who locked people into adult-sized cribs so often that the restraining device was named the Utica Crib. It was invented in the Utica State Lunatic Asylum. People in the field of psychiatry have state power over other people they assign a psychiatric label, and still have no biological evidence of any single claim against them. In their diagnostic manual (Diagnostic and Statistical Manual-V), patient protest forms part of the evidence for the existence of psychiatric disorder, often called anosognosia.

The psychiatric survivor movement operates in a world where racism and discriminations of all types exist. White skin privileges exist. Sex and gender privileges exist. Religious and spiritual privileges exist. A culmination of multiple forms of oppression leaves some in society without power while those who exhibit supremacism maintain power. Rape, for example, is usually about power not about sex, except when rape is about sex that only the aggressor wants, and then rape is categorically about power.

Let's be clear, because someone has been locked up in a psychiatric institution does not mean that they are not racist, or that they are racist, or that they benefit from the realities of racism, or that they have extra burdens due to experienced racism and oppression. Many people who find themselves involved with people in the field of psychology experience hatred and other forms of discrimination that lead to oppression. Often the catalyst for involvement with psychology is the experience of oppression otherwise named with, and masked by, fraudulent psychiatric labels.

Some people in the psychiatric survivor movement like many other movements have understood that the experience of psychiatric oppression is intensified if someone experiences other forms of oppression (see Chapters 7, 12 and 13 in this volume for more on intersectionality). The psychiatric survivor movement I am involved with, sadly, is small these days. We actively seek further involvement of Black, Indigenous, and People of Colour. The psychiatric survivor movement actively seek out ways to include people who experience oppression and discrimination.

The Declaration of Principles, adopted at the 10th Annual Conference Against Psychiatric Oppression and on Human Rights in Toronto, Canada, in 1982, has consistently called for an end of discrimination and inclusion of People of Colour in leadership roles in a movement that has been in a fledgling state for decades, and as will be discussed in this chapter, has fought to exist for centuries.

The peer industry in the US exists. The Substance Abuse and Mental Health Services Administration (2018) published 2017 Data on Mental Health Treatment Facilities offering specific services and practices, by facility type and 'Consumer-run (peer support services)' was one category of programme type analysed. Out of 11,582 total number of facilities, 2,849, or about a quarter of all facilities, offered peer support services (p. 44). An August 2019 report shows 37% of responding facilities offer peer support services (University of Michigan Behavioral Health Workforce Research Center, 2019, 8). I have not been able to find readily available data on the peer support workforce, nationally. In a *National survey of compensation among peer support specialists* (Daniels et al., 2016, 1–37) the category of race is never presented. It is not clear why there are no data for the categories of race and ethnicity in this national survey. Gender is addressed and since this is directly tied to compensation, it is concerning that race and ethnicity are not discussed.

I turn to the network's *Surviving race: The intersection of injustice, disability, and human rights* for greater discussions about modern efforts to address issues of racism within the psychiatric survivor movement and the peer industry. I hope you will also turn to *Surviving race* and get involved (Surviving Race, 2020).

Racism in the field of psychology, however, is the overall issue here and how, at great profit, psy has benefited from the exploitation of people within its grasp. If we trace back through the 19th century, we can see how in the US the discipline of psychology emerged with the reorganisation of the American Psychiatric Association. Medical doctors via the American Psychiatric Association became more particular about who could be part of their trade organisation, newly named as such in 1921. Earlier the American Medico-Psychological Association (established 1892), the real fight between medical doctors and doctors of philosophy took place as non-medical doctors snuck their way in to the Association of Medical Superintendents of American Insane Institutions (established 1844), as a way to strong arm the state and control and dictate the use of taxpayer resources.

The American Psychological Association formed in 1892, the same year as the American Medico-Psychological Association not due to coincidence, but due to the blockage of non-medical doctors wanting entry into what eventually became the American Psychiatric Association. The early divisions between psychiatry and psychology can also be positioned as attempts to be considered legitimate medical practices, and consequent efforts of the medical doctors to bar entry to non-medical practitioners.

From the inception of the Association of Medical Superintendents of American Insane Institutions, issues of race were addressed. For example, the committee on 'On Asylums for Colored Persons' (Curwen, 1885) was established at the first meeting of AMSAII in 1844.

It is hard to imagine that it was only in the mid-1990s that the Office of Ethnic and Minority Affairs of the American Psychological Association established specific work on what racism is, how it exists within psychology, and ways to promote antiracist experiences, and at least to have had an annotated bibliography of the ways in which psychology has been involved in perpetrating racism was important (Office of Ethnic and Minority Affairs, 1998).

Historical racism

Psychiatry, since its inception, has held a tremendous amount of power within American society. Vanessa Jackson (2001) exposed the roles of Benjamin Rush, MD, a signatory to the Declaration of Independence, and Doctor Samuel Cartwright, in the establishment of the practices of scientific racism and the roles of doctors promoting and maintaining systems of slavery and segregation in 19th-century America. Jackson pointed to the creation of psychiatric diagnoses specific to those enslaved and exhibited via the desire for freedom and noncompliance with orders. These so-called symptoms were considered grounds for whipping as cure and prevention.

People get very offended when I say that, when the person enslaving someone could no longer control the person they were trying to enslave, they turned to the alienist/mad doctor/physician/psychiatrist. These medical authorities had (eventually) created segregated institutions where they would offer their 'treatment' of medically sanctioned whippings, recreating the colonial legal status of the whipper and the whipped within the mad doctor industry. Cartwright supported the medical treatment of 'whipping the devil out of them' as a 'preventive measure against absconding or other bad conduct' (Cartwright, 1851/1967, 709). Cartwright in the most degrading way dismisses people freed and focuses his concern about 'rascality' or what he proposed to be dysesthesia: 'to be like a person half asleep, that is with difficulty aroused and kept awake' (p. 710). Concerning those actively enslaved, he says, 'The disease is the natural offspring of negro liberty – the liberty to be idle, to wallow in filth, and to indulge in improper food and drinks' (p. 710). After explaining the supposed disease (drapetomania) that causes people enslaved to not behave the way those enslaving them wanted them to, Cartwright offers the foundational problem and the 'physiological' cure:

> The skin is dry, thick and harsh to the touch, and the liver inactive. The liver, skin and kidneys should be stimulated to activity, and be made to assist in decarbonising the blood. The best means to stimulate the skin is, first, to have the patient well washed with warm water and soap; then, to anoint it all over with oil, and to slap the oil in with a broad leather strap; then to put the patient to some hard kind of work in the open air and sunshine, … any kind of labor will do that … No sooner does the blood feel the vivifying influences … the negro seems to be awakened to a new existence, and to look grateful and thankful to the white man whose compulsory power, has restored his sensation and dispelled the mist that clouded his intellect.
>
> (p. 712)

For decades psychiatric trade organisation publications, and often the minutes of the American Psychiatric Association, from its inception in 1844 under the auspice of AMSAII forward, included debate about segregated institutions and where treatment of people enslaved ultimately would occur. This had a pronounced dividing line in Virginia, specifically between Dr Galt at the Williamsburg Asylum and Dr Stribling at the Staunton Asylum.

The debate was whether people who were enslaved who supposedly needed treatment for their insanity could be 'treated' in the same buildings as white people (see Chapter 2, this volume, on a similar development in East India Company asylums). Galt, a proponent of integrated institutions, suggested white people would not be able to tell the difference between those enslaved in the institution as 'servants' from those who were enslaved and institutionalised for 'treatment', and since they would be working on the farms and shops, the white people would not know they were even there at the institution. (This mirrors debates over a century later in the UK and US concerning potential 'confusion' for visitors if psychiatric nurses were encouraged to wear their own clothes rather than nurse uniform. See Newnes, 2016.)

Opposition to integrated institutions included ideas that white people would know people of African descent would be there, and the institution for whites would be thought to be belittled by the presence of people who were enslaved. The white supremacy was staunch; people enslaved ought *not* be allowed in the same buildings as the white insane unless as their servants. Segregationists eventually won the battle within AMSAII and the win for Stribling led to the development of segregated institutions throughout the United States in the second half of the 19th century (Jackson, 2005).

People often suggest to me that modern psychiatry either does not know about psychiatry's historical involvement with and promotion of slavery or it avidly makes reparations because modern psychiatry acknowledges the discipline's role and is appalled by that same history. Both statements are false. For example, in the same publication that explained the ways possession is considered by contemporary psychiatry to have culturally specific criteria, there is an undated presentation on the DSM-V (Nuckols, n.d.). The presentation starts in the 1840s with the following point then jumps to the 1880s, without any retraction of fact or written acknowledgement of the heinous realities of a) slavery and b) drapetomania:

> 1840 1 DX – US Census – Idiocy/Insanity – Also in the 1840s, southern alienists discovered a malady called Drapetomania – the inexplicable mad longing of a slave for freedom.
>
> (p. 2)

Far from 'discovering' the malady, as with any psychiatric label, the alienists – in this case Cartwright again, in 1852 rather than 'the 1840s' – simply invented it. The third edition of Stedman's *Practical Medical Dictionary* published in 1914 still included an entry for *drapetomania*, defined as 'Vagabondage, dromomania; an uncontrollable or insane impulsion to wander.'

Modernity

People who have experienced oppression because of their group identity (Cross & Cross, 2008) as targets of those who are attempting to maintain power by force are familiar with the consequences of this oppression. White supremacy offers an excellent example for the type of structural oppression devised by the oppressor.

King (2016) discussed the core issues of racism and oppression within the psychiatric system and how the historic horrors of slave medicine still obtain. In an analysis, 'Sixth sense – seeing and diagnosing neo-colonial whiteness' he specified how clear it was to see as he was on the prison ride:

> It emerges as the legacy of slavery is transferred to the modern day psychiatric setting of a prison ward, shut in a cell for 23 hours a day of cultural deprivation and dehumanizing experiences, a number written on your shirt. The sixth sense of whiteness develops as an emotional and

> conceptual tool to translate the narratives of the prison psychiatrist, the prison doctor and the prison social worker that reveal a shared consensus through the white computerized cortex.
>
> (pp. 74–75)

It is important to reflect on the current system in terms of human rights violations carried out through court-ordered and coercive forms of state-sponsored psychiatry such as loss of liberty, forced labour, and prevention of personal economic and social development. Staff and the state maintain their own liberties and benefit from their involvement as employees. Understanding our present situation is important because the story of America changes when retold rejecting the authority of psy.

According to a recent article on the American Psychological Association's website, promoting the career path of 'correctional psychologist', it is estimated the US average annual salary for a correctional psychologist is $111,983. According to the US Bureau of Labor Statistics, the median pay for a psychologist in 2019 was $80,370 per year, with 192,300 jobs in 2019. The mean annual wage for a psychiatrist is $220,380.

John M. Grohol, Psy.D. tabulated the 'Top 25 Psychiatric Medications for 2018' and concluded:

> A total of 611,780,251 prescriptions were made for psychiatric medications in the U.S. in 2018, at a cost of over $29 billion. That's up only 2.42% from 2016, when 597,326,489 psychiatric prescriptions were made.

In the most recent data published by the New York State Office of Mental Health, as of August 12, 2020, in New York City, 22% of people who have Assertive Community Treatment teams assigned to them are White, 22% are identified as 'Other' and more than half (54%) of people are Black. Under a quarter of people (23%) are 'Hispanic'. At a state-wide level, 36% of people are White, 46% of people are Black, and 17% of people described as 'other.' 18% report ethnicity as 'Hispanic' (New York State Office of Mental Health (2020a).

The Assertive Community Treatment programme is one of the most coercive and intrusive psychiatric surveillance programmes coordinated by New York State. It utilises the Assertive Community Treatment model, where members of a treatment team can enter any sphere of a person's life, in their work, school, play or home spaces, to 'check-up' on them. This opens the door for police involvement, and we know, conservatively, one in four police shootings involve the killing of someone who has a psychiatric history (Office of Research and Public Affairs. Treatment Advocacy Center, 2015). The supposed purpose is to ensure that a person is complying with their treatment plan. Treatment plans include products, procedures and programmes a person must comply with to remain in the community to avoid being subjected to court-ordered institutionalisation. Members of gangs called Assertive Community Treatment Teams determine what drugs the person takes, where they are living, what they are eating, how sanitised/organised their home is, how they act or do not act toward or with others, whether or not they socialise enough, or too much.

Of 6,674 people currently in the programme, 65% are male and 35% are female. The average age is 45 years; 6% of people are 24 and younger, 48% 25 to 44, 38% 45 to 64 years old and 8% are 65 or older. Just over one-third (35%) of people have less than a High School Diploma, one-third (33%) of people have a High School Diploma or equivalent, and 23% have some college experience or degree; 9% of people are not accounted for in the data. Only 7% of people are currently employed. The median length of time under an Assertive Community Treatment Team is 2.4 years, with 9% recorded as less than six months and 12% six months to one year. Over one-third (37%) of people are under the programme from one to three years; 17% of people are under a team for three to five years and a quarter (26%) of people under Assertive Community Treatment Teams are subjected to the team's involvement in their life for five or more years. Just over one-fifth (22%) of people in the Assertive Community Treatment programme are under court-ordered Assisted Outpatient Treatment, known as Kendra's Law (New York State Office of Mental Health, 2020b).

Analyses of how psychiatric oppression is greater when other forms of racial, economic and gender oppression exist have been made and have been the subject of consideration as New York's Kendra's Law continues to be challenged, still within a potential sunset period prior to becoming permanently etched into Mental Hygiene Law, with expenditures exceeding $32 million a year.

In addition to involuntary outpatient commitment being an assault on and targeting people who are living in or near poverty, the statistics demonstrate racial disparities – gross overrepresentation of people who are African American – in the application of involuntary outpatient commitment. In the competitive study that was awarded to Swartz et al. (2009) by New York State, commonly referred to as the Duke Study, the authors explain:

> We find that the overrepresentation of African Americans in the AOT Program is a function of African Americans' higher likelihood of being poor, higher likelihood of being uninsured, higher likelihood of being treated by the public mental health system (rather than by private mental health professionals), and higher likelihood of having a history of psychiatric hospitalization. The underlying reasons for these differences in the status of African Americans are beyond the scope of this report.

Staggering racial disparities were documented in the report by Swartz et al. (2009):

> Thus, overall, African Americans are more likely than whites to receive AOT. However, candidates for AOT are largely drawn from a population where blacks are over represented: psychiatric patients with multiple involuntary

> hospitalizations in public facilities. The answer to the question of whether AOT is being applied fairly must take into account all of the available data.

A decade ago, Swartz, et al. (2009) confirmed:

> Since 1999 about 34% of AOT recipients have been African Americans who make up only 17% of the state's population, while 34% of the people on AOT have been whites, who make up 61% of the population.

A decade later, as of 6 September 2020, the Office of Mental Health's statistics show that state-wide, 31% of people under Involuntary Outpatient Commitment and mandated to AOT are White; 37% are Black; 27% are Latinx; 4% are Asian and 1%, Other. So the disparities have grown in the last decade, more people who are Black are court ordered and less people who are White are court ordered. In New York City, Whites drop to less than one-fifth, or 17% of those under court order, people who are Black, skyrocket to nearly half of those court ordered (44%) and people who are Latinx rise to one-third of those mandated to involuntary outpatient treatment, or 33%, of people. The proportion of people who are Asian and committed to community services rises to 6%, and people who identify as 'other' remains at 1%.

Data published by the New York State Office of Mental Health give an indication of who is being subjected to court-ordered psychiatry while living in the community. State-wide, as of 6 September 2020, there have been 43,588 investigations conducted since 1999, 21,833 in New York City. Since 1999, 29,056 petitions have been filed, with 27,709 of the petitions, or 95% of petitions granted. In the period from 6 September 2019 through to 5 September 2020 there were 1,446 petitions filed and 1,289 petitions granted, or 89% of petitions granted. For those who have escaped a court order there was still investigation and involvement with psychiatry in needing to defend their choices, thoughts and actions via psychiatric assessment.

Since 1999, 18,118 people have been under court-ordered psychiatry while living in the community, outside of the walls of the institution, nearly 11,190 of them residing in New York City. This means thousands of people are living under the threat of re-institutionalisation at any moment for noncompliance with the treatment ordered.

State-wide, the average age of people under court order is 38.8 years old. Two-thirds of people under court order are male, one-third are female. People who are of Trans experience or Androgynous or Intersexed are not represented in the data and it is not clear whether or not they are even counted. Three-quarters (75%) of people are single, 4% married, 1% 'cohabiting with significant other', 11% are divorced, 1% are widowed, and the relationship status of 7% of people under court-ordered psychiatry is unknown.

As of 6 August 2020, 2,997 people are under an active court order in New York State. There have been 19,746 people state-wide who have taken the route of supposed 'service enhancements and/or voluntary agreements', with 259 people under this arrangement between August 2019 and July 2020. State-wide, 14,313 people, or 54% of people have been subjected to a renewed order, during the period 6 September 2019 through to 5 September 2020, 876 people, or 57% of people under court order had the order renewed prior to its expiration. Since 1999, the proportion of people under court order that is currently tracked includes 13% of people under court order up to six months, 21% of people six to 12 months; 15% of people have been under the order for 12 to 18 months while 21% of people have been under the order 18 to 30 months. Nearly one-third (30%) of people have been under court order for over 30 months. It is important to keep in mind that these numbers will continue to grow over time; and current orders have the capacity to be renewed.

One of the only ways to get out of the Assisted Outpatient Treatment programme is not an attractive option: re-institutionalisation. During the 12 months ending 5 September 2020, 1,314 people, or 21% of people under court order, were institutionalised. Less than half of people (48%) under court order escape a court order renewal because the criteria for renewal are not met; 4% move out of state and only in 1% of the cases was the renewal of the petition not granted by the court.

Over-representation of people who are African American under Assisted Outpatient Treatment extends to over-representation of People of Colour in nearly all of the involuntary or heavy-surveillance programmes that the New York State Office of Mental Health administers, oversees and evaluates. Notably, and further accentuating racial disparity and economic status, there is under-representation of People of Colour in voluntary psychiatric services. The over-representation of People of Colour in psychiatric programming that utilises force (and limits if not completely eliminates opportunities for economic development for those individuals subject to it) while benefiting those staff of the programme, the State with enhanced budgets via taxpayer resources and the industries that are fuelled by psychiatry, not limited to psychiatric drug industries and device manufacturers, further contextualises the argument that psychiatric inmates (inside or outside of the walls of an institution) are enslaved by psychiatry and why modern psychiatric slavery must be abolished (see Szasz, 1998/1977).

The fact that the United States of America has a long and deeply disturbing history of enacting systems of slavery begs the question of the legitimacy of court-ordered psychiatry, which Swartz et al. (2009) did not answer, but positioned in this way:

> whether AOT is generally seen as beneficial or detrimental to recipients and whether AOT is viewed as a positive mechanism to reduce involuntary hospitalization and improve access to community treatment for an under-served population, or as a program that merely subjects an already-disadvantaged group to a further loss of civil liberties.

This is the context for this work. Psy and particularly court-ordered psy is not only 'a program that merely subjects an already-disadvantaged group to a further loss of civil liberties'. The legitimacy of the court's power for psychiatry suggests that psy must provide legitimate answers to legitimate diseases. However, the entire field of psy rests on the idea of science with no actual biological proof for any disease it identifies and a tremendous amount of data showing the injurious harm and death that treatments have the potential to cause (see Wolfensberger, 1987, on death-making).

The development of the asylum system in the 19th century repositioned as an attempted solution, as social control of those who could not be charged with a crime, allowed for slavery as a form of punishment via the Thirteenth Amendment. If we see the asylum system being built adjacent to the prison complex in the 19th century, we find a story that offers the ways in which the United States government using taxpayer resources, allowed for the continuation of slavery, by another name, via psychiatry, with psychology operating right along in stride.

What you cannot say you cannot abolish

We cannot forget for a moment that the overwhelming majority of people who are subjected to forced/court-ordered psychiatry are People of Colour. Overwhelmingly, people who are of African descent are subjected to court-ordered psychiatry both in institutions and in institutions without walls, in court-ordered involuntary community 'treatment'.

Institutional and structural racism are at the base of this alarming problem. Yes, people need to heal from the legacy of slavery. Yes, psychiatric slavery is different than slavery that the United States was built on, and that needs to be acknowledged. However, as the legal definition of slavery changed from that period, with the establishment of the Thirteenth Amendment legalising slavery for a crime duly committed, we have to deal with the consequences of that change. Psychiatry, certainly inside prisons, but also in its very own institutions, is implicated as the replacement system of slavery, where it would be legal, as a punishment for a duly convicted crime.

We need to be able to deal with the reality that slavery has not been abolished. Slavery has maintained itself as an institution in modern times, through many venues and procedures. The fact that People of Colour are over-represented in court-ordered psychiatry ought to be a concern for all people. It ought to be called what it is, a form of modern slavery for all who are subjected to it – and abolished.

The asylum system has worked in silent tandem with the prison industry under the Thirteenth Amendment, with the exception that no crime need be committed to be put to labour, instead, calling forced labour treatment, under the model of moral treatment.

Elam Lynds was commissioned to build Sing Sing Prison and did it with the labour of people convicted to live in the institution. He marched them down from Auburn, New York, to Ossining, New York, after being forced to resign as overseer for being too harsh on inmates. Lynds was then brought in as the third commissioner of the Utica State Lunatic Asylum, overseeing its completion, and ultimately, eliminating much of its design. He was fired for incompetence by Governor William H. Seward, who eventually became the Secretary of State under Lincoln, because his abolitionist stance was too radical to win the nomination for the presidential run. Seward was wounded in the plot to assassinate Lincoln. In under a decade, Sing Sing was to become one of the legal places slavery was coordinated, and the Utica Asylum, with its dedicated shops and eventual purchase of farms, served the same agenda.

Dix introduced the Ten Million Acre Bill in 1850 at the same time that the Kansas-Nebraska Bill was promoted. Dix, a southern sympathiser, largely credited for the establishment of corporate and state lunatic asylums in the United States, is also credited for helping to start the Civil War, during which she also was a coordinator of nurses; Dix's Nurses, known for caring for injured confederate soldiers (Muckenhoupt, 2003).

Captain John Brown was captured by Robert E. Lee for acts at Harpers Ferry in 1859 with a check from Gerrit Smith in his pocket. Thoreau writes a plea for Brown – Brown refuses the insanity defence. Gerrit Smith is institutionalised at the Utica State lunatic Asylum. John P. Grey MD is Smith's mad doctor. Brown was executed and Smith institutionalised, remaining under psychiatric care the rest of his life – an excellent example of how the prison and asylum system operated in tandem prior to the establishment of the Thirteenth Amendment.

Dr Grey was later shot by Remshaw for opposing testimony given by mad doctor, Isaac Ray. In this court hearing on supposed insanity, Grey was the alienist on behalf of the State for the prosecution of Charles Julius Guiteau's shooting of President Garfield in 1881. Grey refused to acknowledge Guiteau as criminally insane, just as he refused to acknowledge William Spiers, one of the first identified 'rational maniacs' discussed in the *Journal of Insanity* for decades. Grey was Spiers' mad doctor, who took away his keys, causing him to set the Utica State Lunatic Asylum ablaze on Bastille Day, 14 July 1857. Remshaw shot Grey and was sent to the newly minted Marcy State Hospital, for long-term institutionalisation of people deemed unsuccessful at the Utica State Lunatic Asylum, and fated to never again see the light of day.

Slavery is 'one man having absolute power over the life, liberty, and fortune of another' (Black, 1990, 1388). Slavery is ongoing. The Thirteenth Amendment does not eliminate slavery. The Thirteenth Amendment carves out space for who can be legally held in slavery.

> AMENDMENT XIII
>
> Passed by Congress January 31, 1865. Ratified December 6, 1865.
>
> Section 1.
>
> Neither slavery nor involuntary servitude, except as a punishment for crime whereof the party shall have been duly convicted, shall exist within the United States, or any place subject to their jurisdiction.

The institutions of psy and slavery have a long relationship (Jackson, 2001). Two diseases Cartwright details are particularly troubling: Drapetomania and Dysaesthesia Aethiopica. As noted earlier, Drapetomania was a disease of the mind that supposedly caused people enslaved to run away. Symptoms of Drapetomania included a 'sulky disposition and dissatisfying behavior' (Jackson, 2001, 4–5). Cartwright (1851/1967, 707–709) created the disease of someone enslaved wanting to be free one year after Congress passed the Fugitive Slave Act of 1850. The first Fugitive Slave Act had appeared more than a half century before in 1793. Barely six years later mad doctor Benjamin Rush warned of the desire for freedom of people enslaved and wrote of people of African descent, 'they are easily governed' when well cared for and that they must always be oppressed, subservient, 'treated like children', and 'punished until they fall into that submissive state which it was intended for them to occupy' (p. 709).

All of this says Cartwright is to 'prevent and cure them [Slaves] from running away' (p. 709). On 18 September 1850, the Fugitive Slave Act was passed by Congress.

The state-sponsored organised psychiatric industry enacts and benefits from multiple forms of modern slavery. A portion of modern slave labour is not labour in terms of production, but rather, it is labour in terms of consumption. Consumption of drugs which are then billed to the taxpayer and the profits received by the pharmaceutical industry in the form of trillions or more dollars annually, sometimes for *one* drug. The new labour of this type of slavery includes being forced to take the drugs, particularly under court order or compulsion.

The practices, products and procedures supported by large swathes of the fields of psychiatry and psychology routinely cause harm to those who the disciplines assign as in need of their wares. Since before the inception of the fields of psychiatry and psychology, the spiritual experiences of people were psychiatrised and early alienists offered a 'moral treatment' model that sometimes relied on religiosity and other times relied on forced labour. This was also known as a system of slavery where one's life, liberty, and fortune were under the control of another.

Avoiding a recapitulation of oppression

Stockholm Syndrome was named after the discovery that kidnapped and incarcerated people came to 'love' their oppressors. In similar vein, it has been suggested that oppressed people can simply mimic and pass on the act of oppression. In the context of a racist society that oppression may involve imitating racism. As noted at the beginning of this chapter, the psychiatric survivor movement I am involved is small these days. We continue to seek further involvement of Black, Indigenous, and People of Colour.

Since the 10th Annual Conference Against Psychiatric Oppression and on Human Rights in Toronto, Canada, almost 40 years ago, the movement has sought inclusion of People of Colour in leadership roles.

Daniels and colleagues (2016) did not report race and ethnicity as categories in national surveys of peer support. If the movement is not to mimic the racist oppression endemic in psy it is essential that any potential challenge is not rendered invisible through a lack of data.

It is my understanding that, due to my asking questions about these data, a National Survey to assess representation of Black, Indigenous, and People of Colour (BIPOC) in the peer industry is being developed. I believe the survey ought to include questions about their perspectives about forced treatment, if and how their advocacy is used in the processes of forced treatment, and any forced or subsequent unwanted involvement they have with the psy industries or discrimination they experience because of their employed role as a 'peer'.

It is worth repeating that the network's *Surviving race: The intersection of injustice, disability, and human rights* can act as a basis for discussion about modern efforts to address issues of racism within the psychiatric survivor movement and the peer industry. Read *Surviving race*. Get involved.

References

Asylum log (2020). *Utica State Lunatic Asylum Managers Log*, 1844 www.facebook.com/theasylumlog/ Accessed 10 October 2020.

Black, H. C. (1990). *Black's law dictionary: Definitions of the terms and phrases of American and English jurisprudence, ancient and modern*. St. Paul, MN: West Publishing Co.

Cartwright, S. (1851/1967). Diseases and peculiarities of the Negro race. *De Bow's Review Southern and Western States* 11, New Orleans. Reprinted: New York: AMS Press.

Chamberlin, J. (1990). The ex-patients' movement: Where we've been and where we're going. *Journal of Mind and Behavior, 11*, 323–336.

Cross, W. E., Jr. (1971). The Negro to Black conversion experience: Toward a psychology of Black liberation. *Black World, 20*, 13–27.

Cross, W. E., Jr., & Cross, T. B. (2008). The big picture: Theorizing self-concept structure and construal. In P. Peredsen et al. (Eds.). *Counseling across Cultures* (6th ed., pp. 73–88). Thousand Oaks, CA: Sage Press.

Curwen, J. (1885). *History of the Association of Medical Superintendents of American Institutions for the Insane from 1844 to 1884, inclusive, with a list of the different hospitals for the insane, and the names and dates of appointment and resignation of the medical superintendents*. Warren, PA: F. Cowan.

Daniels, A. S., Ashenden, P., Goodale, L., & Stevens, T. (2016). *National survey of compensation among peer support specialists*. The College for Behavioral Health Leadership, www.acmha.org, January, 2016. https://papeersupportcoalition.org/wp-content/uploads/2016/01/CPS_Compensation_Report.pdf. Accessed 23 January 2016.

Geller, J., & Harris, M. (1994). *Women of the asylum. (For Elizabeth Stone; Elizabeth Packard; Phylis Chesler; and Phebe Davis)*. New York: Doubleday.

Goffman, E. (1961). *Asylums: Essays on the social situations of mental patients and other inmates*. New York: Doubleday.

Goffman, E. (1963). *Stigma: Notes on the management of spoiled identity*. New York: Prentice Hall.

Grohol, J. M. (2018). Top 25 psychiatric medications for 2018. https://psychcentral.com/blog/top-25-psychiatric-medications-for-2018/. Accessed 23 January 2020.

Jackson, V. (2001). *In our own voice: African-American stories of oppression, survival, and recovery in mental health systems. It's about time: Discovering, recovering and celebrating mental health consumer/survivor history*. www.healingcircles.org/uploads/2/1/4/8/2148953/inovweb.pdf. Accessed 22 February 2014.

Jackson, V. (2005). *Separate and unequal: The legacy of racially segregated psychiatric hospitals. A cultural competence training tool*. Monograph. www.healingcircles.org/uploads/2/1/4/8/2148953/sauweb.pdf.

Jackson, V. (2008). In our own voice: African American perspectives on mental health. Program related to the exhibition, 'The lives they left behind: Suitcases from a state hospital attic.' On view at the Science, Industry, and Business Library from 3 December 2007 to 31 January 2008.

King, C. (2016). Whiteness in psychiatry: The madness of European misdiagnosis In. J. Russo, & A. Sweeney (Eds.). *Searching for a rose garden: Challenging psychiatry, fostering mad studies*. Monmouth: PCCS Books.

Muckenhoupt, M. (2003). *Dorothea Dix: Advocate for mental health care*. Oxford: Oxford University Press.

New York State Office of Mental Health. (2020a). Assisted outpatient treatment: program statistics. https://my.omh.ny.gov/analytics/saw.dll?PortalPages&PortalPath=%2Fshared%2FAOTLP%2F_portal%2FAssisted%20Outpatient%20Treatment%20Reports&Page=home#reports. Accessed 6 September 2020.

New York State Office of Mental Health. (2020b). Assertive community treatment data. https://omh.ny.gov/omhweb/tableau/act.html. Accessed 6 September 2020.

Newnes, C. (2016). *Inscription, diagnosis and deception in the mental health industry: How psy governs us all*. Basingstoke: Palgrave Macmillan.

Nuckols, C. (n.d.). www.google.co.uk/search?sxsrf=ALeKk03J6el_fjg-qoSr1Dht85u45TBFnQ:1600256007793&source=univ&tbm=isch&q=DHSS+Delaware+government+website,+Presentation+on+DSM+5+by+Nuckols&sa=X&ved=2ahUKEwjqjJOXyu3rAhUMAcAKHQtfA2sQ7Al6BAgKEB4&biw=1517&bih=730#imgrc=dpq-thuxoltyFM. Accessed 14 September 2020.

Office of Ethnic Minority Affairs, American Psychological Association. (March 1998). *Annotated bibliography of psychology and racism*. www.apa.org/pi/oema/resources/brochures/race-biblio. Accessed 3 October 2020.

Office of Research and Public Affairs. Treatment Advocacy Center. (December 2015). *Overlooked in the undercounted: The role of mental illness in law enforcement encounters*. www.treatmentadvocacycenter.org/storage/documents/overlooked-in-the-undercounted.pdf. Accessed 11 October 2020.

Stinger, H. (2020). Careers in corrections. *Monitor on Psychology, 51*(2), March. Print version: page 62. www.apa.org/monitor/2020/03/careers-corrections. Accessed 5 October 2020.

Substance Abuse and Mental Health Services Administration, National Mental Health Services Survey (N-MHSS) (2017). Data on mental health treatment facilities. Rockville, MD: Substance abuse and mental health services administration, 2018. Table 2.4a. Mental health treatment facilities offering specific services and practices, by facility type: Number, 2017. www.samhsa.gov/data/sites/default/files/cbhsq-reports/2017_National_Mental_Health_Services_Survey.pdf. Accessed5 August 2019.

Surviving Race (2020). www.facebook.com/groups/364074427086419/ Accessed 4 October 2020.

Swartz, M.S, Swanson, J.W., Steadman, H.J., Robbins, P.C., & Monahan J. (2009). *New York State Assisted Outpatient Treatment program evaluation*. Durham, NC: Duke University School of Medicine.

Szasz, T. (1998/1977). *Psychiatric slavery*. New York: Syracuse University Press.

Szasz, T. (2002). *Liberation by oppression: A comparative study of slavery and psychiatry*. New Brunswick, NJ: Transaction Publishers.

Tenney, L. (2006). Who fancies to have a Revolution here? The Opal Revisited (1851–1860). *Journal of Radial Psychology, 5*. www.radpsynet.org/journal/vol5/Tenney.html. Accessed 14 October 2008.

Tenney, L. J. (2008). Psychiatric slave no more: Parallels to a Black liberation psychology. *Journal of Radical Psychology*. 7(1), 2–11. www.radicalpsychology.org/vol7-1/tenney2008.html. Accessed 14 February 2014.

Tenney, L. J. (2014). (de)VOICED: Human rights now. VI, II, and III. Dissertation. PhD Program in Environmental Psychology. Proquest.

United States of America. (1794-1992). *Constitution of the United States*. National Archives. www.archives.gov/founding-docs/amendments-11–27. Accessed 5 October 2020.

University of Michigan Behavioral Health Workforce Research Center. (2019). *National analysis of peer support providers: Practice settings, requirements, roles, and reimbursements*. Ann Arbor, MI: UMSPH. www.behavioralhealthworkforce.org/wp-content/uploads/2019/10/BHWRC-Peer-Workforce-Full-Report.pdf. Retrieved. 5 October 2020.

Wolfensberger, W. (1987). *The new genocide of handicapped and afflicted people*. New York: University of Syracuse.

Part II

Race, theory and practice

Chapter 7

Racism and learning disabilities

Deborah Chinn

Summary

This chapter started life as a short paper published in *Clinical Psychology Forum* in 2018, which I was then invited to present at the 2019 annual conference for the British Psychological Society (BPS) Division of Clinical Psychology (DCP) as part of a symposium on Racism, Psychology and Invisibility brought together by Craig Newnes. The choice of the last word – 'invisibility' – reflected the frustration that I and others presenting at the symposium felt at the reluctance at naming racism as a force experienced by our service users, in my case service users with learning disabilities and their families and supporters, and ever present in the institutions where we worked.

Since the Summer of 2020, racism is appearing front and centre in public debate.[1] Incontrovertible evidence emerged about the disproportionate death rate amongst BAME citizens from COVID-19 in the UK and US, at least in part because of a disregard for their safety as key workers working in care roles, transport and retail, and most likely to be dangerously exposed to the virus. The shocking death of George Floyd in the US reignited anger across the world at police brutality targeting people of colour and highlighted the inescapability of systems of oppression for Black people that lead to exclusion, disempowerment and even death. This feels like the right moment to take a closer look at how racism plays out in the lives of people with learning disabilities and those who support them.

In this chapter I explore the origins of our professional technologies as clinical psychologists, and identify how our institutions and practices reinforce widely circulating understandings of racial and ethnic diversity as unvarying and one-dimensional, constructed as deficit and risk. I explore the generally sparse evidence of health and social inequalities experienced by people with learning disabilities from BAME groups. Many people with learning disabilities live in care relationships and their well-being is intimately connected with the well-being of those who support them. I therefore look at how racial discrimination is a force in the lives of family caregivers and support staff. Furthermore, I question whether the strategies we have at the moment can really achieve anti-oppressive practice. The perspective throughout is from the UK learning disability service context, so some arguments and examples are very much linked to this, though others have more general relevance.

In talking about race and disability it is common to use an additive or cumulative metaphor using terms such as 'a double disadvantage'. Instead of this I am going to use the framework of intersectionality, introduced by Kimberle Crenshaw to understand the experiences of black women in the US (Crenshaw, 1989). This framework highlights the way that different aspects of diversity interconnect to bring about qualitatively different experiences because of the ways that oppressive responses to difference (racism, homophobia, sexism, ableism) interact and reinforce each other. Intersectionality also explicitly focuses on how oppressive intersections are organised and how larger historical processes, structural distributions of resources and power and recurring tropes and forms of representation shape the complexity of people's everyday lives. This approach calls explicit attention to how the complexity of people's everyday experiences is connected to larger historical processes, and this is just as true of an individual's experience of disability as it of race.

Technologies of measurement and diagnosis

In considering the intersection of race and disability for people with learning disabilities, we need to reconsider and resist the way that race and disability are institutionalised, as Chen and Mathies (2016, 235) put it, as 'orthogonal in nature to one another rather than con-constitutive'. Race, racism and learning disability are inextricably intertwined in the history of the development of professional psychology. The origin of the Western category of learning disabilities lies in 'race science' – a fundamental belief in genetic determinism, that 'races' are biologically distinct and have different socially prized attributes as a result. The intense interest in differences in intellectual capacity and the systems of categorisation and quantification of 'intelligence' was stimulated by the 19th-century eugenics movement in North America and Western Europe. The same period saw the establishment of the psy professions and their forms of disciplinary knowledge (Foucault, 1977).

In the face of unprecedented movements of peoples – of poor people from southern and eastern Europe, and former slaves within the US, White elites developed the concept of 'feeble mindedness' and other categories of intellectual deficiency, based on a racialised conception of intelligence (Trent, 1994). This was underpinned by a racial hierarchy, with White people at the top, supposedly possessing normal or superior cognitive ability and other races ranged below. The men associated with these ideas, from John Langdon Down to Francis Galton and Karl Pearson, supplied us with terminology (Down's Syndrome) and techniques of quantification and biometry (chi-squared test, standard deviation, correlation coefficients) that underpin clinical psychology practice today. The delineation of learning disabilities as a category relies on

Galton's concept of the norm as a statistical concept that divides the non-standard from the standard sub-population (Davis, 1997). Galton's work made possible the development of the intelligence quotient (IQ) and the measurement and stratification of degrees of 'intelligence' as an individual, stable, unitary psychological property linked to genetic makeup.

Despite decades of criticism and controversy, the IQ test is still used by clinical psychologists to confer learning disability status on people seeking support to negotiate the challenges of modern life. Its reliance on an underpinning contention that there is such a thing as biologically based 'general intelligence', however vaguely described, goes largely unchallenged. The IQ test is commonly described as a tool for 'diagnosis' of learning disabilities, as if this category was analogous to a physical illness that can be detected using the appropriate technology, used by specially trained experts in the field. This is despite tacit acceptance in many quarters, including the British Psychological Society, that learning disabilities are more helpfully understood as a historically and culturally specific social construction, and that IQ tests have many flaws and are of doubtful reliability and validity for individuals who have not grown up in English language environments and have had limited experience of the UK culture and education system.

Webb & Whitaker (2012) describe the double think employed by many clinical psychologists, privately acknowledging the limitations of IQ tests and the arbitrary nature of the cut-off score of 70 IQ points that defines learning disability, whilst publicly and professionally talking about learning disabilities as 'as if it were a real, naturally occurring condition' (p. 440). Thus the diagnostic procedure involving IQ tests can be seen as a way of passing off culturally specific norms of competence (measured through arcane rituals of assessment) as if they were universal and incontrovertible.

Despite being discredited repeatedly, 'race science' refuses to die. It has proved to be a slippery adversary, with the capacity to lurk in academic and political discourse. A more up-to-date term, hereditarianism, disguises adherence to the principles of scientific racism. Its more egregious and flamboyant proponents have been 'named and shamed' for frankly racist comments, though despite this, a number of these proponents such as James Watson, Chris Brand, Phillipe Rushton and Richard Lynn, have occupied prestigious academic positions. Spokespeople for the 'new geneism' adopt a 'softly softly' approach (Gillborn, 2016) avoiding any mention of race, despite a reliance on a fundamental assumption that racial inequity is genetically shaped, ignoring the impact of structural social inequality (Duster, 2003). The premise that variations in achievement evidenced by different social groups is a simple fact of life that should be supported by educational and social policy is bolstered by association with politicians at the highest level. The UK Prime Minister Boris Johnson has justified selective education privileging those with higher IQ scores and his closest political adviser Dominic Cummings then publicly attributed variation in achievements of school children largely to genetic factors (Gillborn, 2016).

BAME people with learning disabilities and health and social inequalities

In expanding my original article I found myself searching repeatedly for up-to-date research that specifically explored health and social inequalities and inequities experienced by people with learning disabilities from BAME groups; finding such data was very difficult in many areas. 'Learning disability' as an attribute represented in research, policy and practice is characterised as a 'master category'; a set of individual deficits that perturb everyday life to such a fundamental extent that all other categories to which the individual may belong are deemed secondary. Learning disability is constructed as deficit, tragedy and burden, leaving little space for the individual to engage in social life as a person who can claim a sexual, ethnic and indeed a political identity. Commonly, researchers either neglect to include ethnicity as a variable, make few efforts to create diverse samples representative of local communities, or fail to explore and explain differences between BAME and White groups (Jones, 2001). Robertson et al. (2019) recently undertook a systematic review of health and healthcare of people with learning disabilities from minority ethnic groups in the UK and made the same observation – 'little is known', particularly about physical health outcomes. This is itself a barrier to anti-racist practice; unless we can identify disparities in experiences or outcomes relating to ethnicity we cannot begin to rectify them.

The Robertson et al. (2019) review and an earlier one by Durà-Vilà & Hodes (2012) do provide some insights on disparities between ethnic groups in health service utilisation and health outcomes. Most of the research cited relates to mental health and specialist learning disability services. Both sets of authors noted the preponderance of research into the experiences of people from South Asian backgrounds, partly because of the pioneering work of psychologists and psychiatrists of South Asian heritage, particularly those in Leicester, UK. Whilst celebrating the work of BAME researchers, we should also recognise the extra burden they face in personally having to negotiate racism as researchers (Maylor, 2009). Doing research on racism and discrimination is everyone's business even if the academic and practitioner audience would rather look the other way (Parker, 1997).

The research evidence available on healthcare disparities among BAME people with learning disabilities emphasises barriers to service use (Durà-Vilà & Hodes, 2012; Robertson et al., 2019). Service recipients from BAME communities make less use of specialist mental health services (Bhaumik et al., 2008; Raghavan & Waseem, 2007) and also report higher levels of unmet needs for health and social care (Devapriam et al., 2008). However, stereotyping of BAME groups mean that service providers fail to address reduced service access among BAME service users, assuming that these families 'look after their own' (Heer et al., 2016; Mir et al., 2001) or are 'hard to reach' – rather than 'easy to ignore' (Johnson, 2008).

A recurring theme is concern among BAME families and service users about lack of cultural appropriateness and cultural sensitivity in services, perceived racism and language barriers. Experience of racism in mental health and other public services among some African-Caribbean communities contributes to realistically founded fears 'that involvement with mental health services could eventually lead to their death' (Keating & Robertson, 2004). Recent policy enforcing a responsibility to monitor service users for signs of radicalisation under the UK counter-terrorism 'Prevent' agenda has led to further worries about the consequences of engagement with public services among Muslim service users (Byrne et al., 2017). BAME families, including those supporting a person with learning disabilities, are therefore at risk of delaying making contact with services before crisis point is reached (Heer et al., 2016).

The shift over the last 20 years towards personalisation in public services (Netten et al., 2012) with the promotion of personal budgets and direct payments has been heralded as creating opportunities for service users and families from BAME groups to select and manage culturally appropriate care (Moriarty, 2014). However, as O'Shaugnessy and Tilki point out 'a feeling that…that attention to individualised care will transcend [cultural differences] can result in discrimination, which although unintentional, potentially constitutes institutional racism' (O'Shaughnessy & Tilki, 2007, 74–75). Service users and families from BAME groups are likely to require input and support from third sector and advocacy services specifically geared to their needs to make best use of personalisation. This support is chronically underfunded and has been further eroded under conditions of austerity politics in UK public services (Fulton & Richardson, 2010; Moriarty, 2014).

In many other contexts where data exist of health and social inequalities experienced by people with learning disabilities and of disparities experienced by people from BAME groups, there is little or no research to integrate the two sets of data or to explain associations if they are found (Jones, 2001). In the COVID-19 pandemic, it is clear that people from BAME groups are experiencing markedly higher rates of mortality from the disease for reasons linked to racism, discrimination and social inequality (Iacobucci, 2020). We also know that deaths among people with learning disabilities have risen at an alarming rate during the pandemic (Lintern, 2020). But as yet we have no information about how the pandemic might be disproportionally affecting people with learning disabilities from BAME groups, either directly or indirectly through loss of family, friends and caregivers.

Moving to a different setting – the overrepresentation of people from some BAME groups in the criminal justice system (CJS) is well established (Williams et al., 2012). There are also data from different sources that around 10% of offenders in contact with the criminal justice system are inscribed with learning disabilities (Hellenbach et al., 2017), with 20–30% classifiable as having 'borderline learning disabilities', leading to the conclusion that 'it is highly likely that people from BAME communities [and learning disabilities] are disproportionately over-represented in the CJS' (Saunders et al., 2013). However, UK research on how learning disabilities and BAME status intersect to create disadvantage within the CJS hardly exists. A study conducted by the Prison Reform Trust involved interviews with 173 prisoners with learning disabilities and learning difficulties, 23% of whom were from BAME groups – compared to 14% in the general UK population (Talbot, 2008). However, consideration of the 'double disadvantage' experienced by this group was not included in the report and was instead earmarked for 'future research'.

Racial discrimination in the learning disability workforce

A further overlooked dimension where racism and discrimination may be affecting the care of people with learning disabilities relates to the make-up of the paid care sector. Of the adult social care workforce 21% are from BAME backgrounds, compared to 14% of the English population (Skills for Care, 2019). In London this figure rises to 67% where 34% of all workers are from BAME groups. A great deal of clinical psychology input in learning disability contexts works through direct care staff as mediators of interventions. Potentially these workers provide a culturally sensitive resource for service users from BAME groups and operate as cultural mediators between these groups and the largely White clinical psychology workforce.

This group of employees experiences disadvantage and discrimination that is often not acknowledged or addressed. Direct care workers are among the lowest paid groups of employees, earning less than £200 per week (Taylor, 2018). Moreover, care workers from BAME groups experience an 'ethnicity pay gap', receiving significantly less pay than White workers in the same sector (Hussein & Manthorpe, 2014). They have to deal with racism from service users and from employers (Stevens et al., 2012). Brown and Smith (1995, 169) emphasised the importance of ensuring 'the utmost care in the language used to describe the people who do the caring and a consistent refusal to scapegoat or blame them'. This guidance needs to be revived and updated with an emphasis on working with and supporting BAME care workers.

Difference, deficit and diversity

I certainly am not the first person to highlight the burden of disadvantage experienced by people with learning disabilities in the UK who are from BAME communities, and I would like to express my appreciation of work done in the past. The importance of culturally sensitive services for people with learning disabilities was emphasised in *Learning Difficulties and Ethnicity: Framework for action* (Valuing People Support Team & Department of Health, 2004), *Valuing People Now* (Department of Health, 2009) and statements from the Division of Clinical Psychology (2011) and the Royal College of Psychiatrists (Gangadharan et al., 2011). These documents contain many relevant and helpful statements about the importance of communicating effectively with service users and their families from BAME groups, using interpreters, and being sensitive to different customs, beliefs and practices.

What is also apparent from these documents is a tendency to focus on 'cultural differences' framed as deficit – lack of proper understanding of what learning disabilities 'means', misconceptions, such as 'searching for a cure' (Gangadharan et al., 2011), lack of awareness and knowledge about services (Valuing People Support Team & Department of Health, 2004), and the risks of consanguineous marriage (see www.towerhamlets.gov.uk/Documents/Borough_statistics/JSNA/Consanguinity-JSNA- Fact-Sheet.pdf for a thoughtful discussion of this issue and some effective myth-busting), lack of language skills, lack of understanding of service goals and philosophies premised on individual autonomy and rights (Moriarty, 2014). Furthermore, we can see how BAME status can be identified, not only as a deficit but also as a risk factor when linked with learning disabilities; for instance, in the context of the UK government Prevent strategy to counter domestic terrorist activities, autism and learning disabilities are frequently cited as risk factors for radicalisation of British Muslims in public commentary on domestic terrorism (Heath-Kelly, 2018), despite little evidence to support this.

These messages can be perceived as stereotyping and stigmatising by people from BAME communities and compound reluctance to engage with services (Hatton et al., 2010). Others have argued that this emphasis on 'cultural differences' to explain health and social inequalities experienced by people from BAME communities overlooks the importance of social and economic marginalisation and racism (Ahmad & Bradby, 2007). Indeed, there seems to be a noticeable discomfort with the concept of racism and the operation of unconscious bias within service and institutional discourses (van Herwaarden et al., 2020), including those of clinical psychology.

Decolonising psychology

The movement to decolonise psychology attempts to displace the dominance of psychologies that have been developed in the global north and, instead of reasserting their scientific truth and universality, sees them as historically and culturally specific (Adams et al., 2015). Decolonising psychology also means making space for psychologies developed by indigenous and majority world peoples and understanding how (in)competence is understood in different cultural setting (Jenkins, 1998). Clinical psychology has been involved in a colonising project, reproducing itself and its institutional values and concepts across the world. Institutions such as the International Association for the Scientific Study of Intellectual and Developmental Disability (IASSIDD) reinforce the messages of what constitute universally legitimate understandings of learning disabilities and appropriate treatments and interventions (Newnes, 2018). Other chapters in this book problematise and denaturalise the focus on individualism, rationalism and autonomous self-management that characterise the neoliberal psychological subject, including the learning-disabled subject of clinical psychology attention. Contrasting understandings of humanity, well-being and difference might emphasise spirituality and connectedness to rhythms and cycles of the natural world and to ancestors (Dudgeon & Walker, 2015) as well as views of mental competence that is socially distributed (rather than an attribute of the individual) (Booth & Booth, 2007); as manifested through compliance with social norms of tractability, civility and conversational ability (Whyte, 1998) or through care and interest in others (Jegatheesan et al., 2010)

Indigenous psychologies may open up opportunities for people with learning disabilities. Our research with people from the Bangladeshi/Sylheti community in the east end of London (Durling et al., 2018) found that community understandings of personhood of people with learning disabilities conferring eligibility for acceptance into the cultural and religious 'cycle of life' included them in institutions of marriage and parenting more commonly denied to people with learning disabilities from white British families. However, there are pitfalls associated with the 'indigenisation project'. The first is romanticisation of minority ethnic communities' responses to disability that can overlook how intersections of disability, racial/ethnic identity in diverse communities can oppress and harm people with learning disabilities, especially when the impact of gender is added to the mix (Mehrotra & Vaidya, 2008).

The second pitfall is that of overgeneralising from local, specific strategies that have legitimacy to particular marginalised communities that may have limited relevance to others and limited ability to present an effective alternative to hegemonic psychological science. For instance, Jegatheesan and colleagues (2010) noted that Muslim parents' conceptualisation of autism as a gift from God, and as a condition that should not stand in the way of their children's full involvement in the life of the community, led to the parents' forthright rejection of professionals' focus on autism as a constellation of social communication deficits. The researchers do not tell us how the parents' voiced this resistance to professionals. If they did, it is likely they would be dismissed as 'in denial' or 'misunderstanding' the true nature of autism.

Superdiversity

A further pitfall of indigenisation is reification and cultural essentialism: the assumption that cultural patterns and concepts are fixed and timeless essences of social groupings, rather than fluid, ecologically responsive and negotiated (Adams et al., 2015). Reification is a pervasive trope within discussions of race and culture in service settings and can shade into oversimplification and stereotyping. Rather than thinking of relatively bounded homogeneous 'communities', the concept of 'superdiversity' attempts to reflect the 'dynamic interplay of variables among an increased number of new, small and scattered, multiple-origin, transnationally connected, socio-economically differentiated and legally stratified immigrants' (Vertovec, 2007).

Superdiversity is a diversification of diversity, brought about by globalisation and new patterns of migration, and the opportunities for the growth of networks of information and sociality created by digital technologies. In sociolinguistics, the concept of superdiversity has stimulated an interest in the way that citizens draw on culturally patterned communicative resources and practices from a range of local subgroups (including their own), as they negotiate their way in a complex and fast-moving urban environment (Arnaut et al., 2016). Ethnic identity is seen as fluid, hybrid and occasioned, more what Goffman would describe as a carefully crafted 'performance' (Goffman, 1959) designed to achieve specific social goals than an intrinsic characteristic of the individual.

We have accounts from young Asian women with learning disabilities about how they negotiate their ethnic identities in these ways (Malik et al., 2017), articulated through their selective use of dietary practices, dress and linguistic registers in different settings. Such nuanced descriptions of 'ethnic identity' relating to people with learning disabilities and their families are rare, and research and policy more often use broad terms such as 'Asian' or 'black British' that oversimplify the individual positions and cultural practices that people adopt.

Institutional ambivalence

Reviewing the progress made by Learning Disability Partnership Boards six years after *Valuing People* (Department of Health, 2001), Chris Hatton found that services were still failing to consider BAME communities when planning learning disability services (Hatton, 2007). More than ten years later, and after a decade of austerity politics, third-sector organisations serving BAME groups, including people with learning disabilities, have seen drastic cuts in funding, and some have been disbanded, including the invaluable Bangladeshi Parent Advisor Service in Tower Hamlets (Davis & Choudhury, 1988) which provided advice and emotional support for Bangladeshi families of people with learning disabilities.

A more recent large-scale initiative in learning disability service provision in the UK, following the Winterbourne scandal that exposed the abuse of people with intellectual disabilities in residential settings, has been the Transforming Care agenda (Bubb, 2014). The guidance and strategy documents supporting Transforming Care contain no specific mention of the needs of BAME services users, or any consideration of how transformed services need to be designed with them in mind. One might conclude that, despite the popularity of the discourses of diversity and inclusion, the requirements of people with learning disabilities and their families from BAME group are not seen as 'core business' for funders of health and social care.

'Institutional ambivalence' might also describe our position as clinical psychologists working with people with learning disabilities from BAME groups. We certainly wish to do better, but are perhaps held back by our reluctance to examine the frankly racist roots of our profession, and our enmeshment in service structures that struggle to both make sense of the complexities and oppressions experienced by people with learning disabilities from BAME communities and to appreciate and make use of the rich understandings of difference they can offer. My own approach here draws from contemporary anti-racist practice fuelled by Black Lives Matter; understanding the systematic and institutionalised discrimination that BAME communities and individuals experience and that Whiteness protects others from. It can take an effort for a White clinical psychologist like myself to 'see' racism in the lives of service users with learning disabilities and indeed in the services set up to support them. I hope this chapter can open up lines for debate and discussion amongst researchers and practitioners and opportunities for the promotion of genuinely anti-racist practice.

Note

1 I use the term 'learning disabilities' in this chapter, rather than other terms in circulation in research literature (intellectual disabilities, developmental disability) as this used is the term in service contexts and in common parlance in the UK. I use the term 'race' not as a genetically determined individual attribute, but as a social category.

References

Adams, G., Dobles, I., Gómez, L. H., Kurtiş, T., & Molina, L. E. (2015). Decolonizing psychological science: Introduction to the special thematic section. *Journal of Social and Political Psychology*, *3*(1), 213–238.

Ahmad, W. I., & Bradby, H. (2007). Locating ethnicity and health: Exploring concepts and contexts. *Sociology of Health and Illness*, *29*(6), 795–810.

Arnaut, K. , Blommaert, J., Rampton, B., & Spotti, M. (Eds.) (2016). *Language and Superdiversity*. London: Routledge.

Bhaumik, S., Tyrer, F. C., McGrother, C., & Ganghadaran, S. K. (2008). Psychiatric service use and psychiatric disorders in adults with intellectual disability. *Journal of Intellectual Disability Research*, *52*(11), 986–995.

Booth, T., & Booth, W. (2007). Parental competence and parents with learning difficulties. *Child and Family Social Work*, *1*(2), 81–86.

Brown, H., & Smith, H. (1992). *Normalisation: A reader*. London: Routledge.

Bubb, S. (2014). *Winterbourne View – time for change: Transforming the commissioning of services for people with learning disabilities and/or autism*. London: HMSO. www.england.nhs.uk/wp-content/uploads/2014/11/transforming-commissioning-services.pdf

Byrne, A., Mustafa, S., & Miah, I. Q. (2017). Working together to break the 'circles of fear'between Muslim communities and mental health services. *Psychoanalytic Psychotherapy*, *31*(4), 393–400.

Chen, P. D., & Mathies, C. (2016). Assessment, evaluation, and research. *New Directions for Higher Education*, *175*, 85–92. https://doi.org/10.1002/he.20202

Crenshaw, K. (1989). Demarginalizing the intersection of race and sex: A Black feminist critique of antidiscrimination doctrine, feminist theory and antiracist politics. *University of Chicago Legal Forum*, article 8. https://chicagounbound.uchicago.edu/uclf/vol1989/iss1/8

Davis, H., & Choudhury, P. A. (1988). Helping Bangladeshi families: Tower Hamlets parent adviser scheme. *British Journal of Learning Disabilities, 16*(2), 48–51.

Davis, L. J. (1997). Constructing normalcy. *The Disability Studies Reader, 3*, 3–19.

Department of Health. (2001). *Valuing people: A new strategy for learning disability for the 21st century*. London: Stationery Office. https://scholar.google.com/scholar?q=Department+of+Health+(2001b)+Valuing+People:+A+New+Strategy+for+Learning+Disability+for+the+21st+Century.+London:+Stationery+Office.

Department of Health. (2009). *Valuing people now. Summary report March2009–September 2010, including findings from Learning Disabiity Partnership Board Self-Assessments 2009–2010*. London: DoH.

Devapriam, J., Thorp, C., Tyrer, F., Gangadharan, S., Raju, L., & Bhaumik, S. (2008). A comparative study of stress and unmet needs in carers of South Asian and white adults with learning disabilities. *Ethnicity and Inequalities in Health and Social Care, 1*(2), 35–43.

Division of Clinical Psychology. (2011). *Guidelines for clinical psychology services*. Leicester: BPS.

Dudgeon, P., & Walker, R. (2015). Decolonising Australian psychology: Discourses, strategies, and practice. *Journal of Social and Political Psychology, 3*(1), 276–297. https://doi.org/10.5964/jspp.v3i1.126

Durà-Vilà, G., & Hodes, M. (2012). Ethnic factors in mental health service utilisation among people with intellectual disability in high-income countries: Systematic review. *Journal of Intellectual Disability Research, 56*(9), 827–842.

Durling, E., Chinn, D., & Scior, K. (2018). Family and community in the lives of UK Bangladeshi parents with intellectual disabilities. *Journal of Applied Research in Intellectual Disabilities, 31*(6), 1133–1143.

Duster, T. (2003). *Backdoor to eugenics*. London: Psychology Press.

Foucault, M. (1977). *Discipline and Punish: The birth of the prison*. New York: Random House.

Fulton, R., & Richardson, K. (2010). Towards race equality in advocacy services: People with learning disabilities from black and minority ethnic communities. *Better Health Brief, 15*, 1–7.

Gangadharan, S. K., Bhaumik, S., Devapriam, J., Hiremath, A., Johnson, M., O'Hara, J., Raghavan, R., Sidat, R., & Surti, Y. (2011). Minority ethics communities and specialist learning disability services: Report of the Faculty of the Psychiatry of Learning Disability Working Group. Newcastle: Royal College of Psychiatrists. http://nrl.northumbria.ac.uk/5944/1/FR_LD_2%20for%20web.pdf

Gillborn, D. (2016). Softly, softly: Genetics, intelligence and the hidden racism of the new geneism. *Journal of Education Policy, 31*(4), 365–388. https://doi.org/10.1080/02680939.2016.1139189

Goffman, E. (1959). *The presentation of self in everyday life*. New York: Doubleday.

Hatton, C. (2007). *Improving services for people with learning disabilities from minority ethnic communities: The second national survey of partnership boards*. Lancaster: Lancaster University. Available at www.etn.leeds.

Hatton, C., Emerson, E., Kirby, S., Kotwal, H., Baines, S., Hutchinson, C., Dobson, C., & Marks, B. (2010). Majority and minority ethnic family carers of adults with intellectual disabilities: Perceptions of challenging behaviour and family impact. *Journal of Applied Research in Intellectual Disabilities, 23*(1), 63–74.

Heath-Kelly, C. (2018). Forgetting ISIS: Enmity, drive and repetition in security discourse. *Critical Studies on Security, 6*(1), 85–99. DOI: 10.1080/21624887.2017.1407595

Heer, K., Rose, J., & Larkin, M. (2016). The challenges of providing culturally competent care within a disability focused team: A phenomenological exploration of staff experiences. *Journal of Transcultural Nursing, 27*(2), 109–116. https://doi.org/10.1177/1043659614526454

Hellenbach, M., Karatzias, T., & Brown, M. (2017). Intellectual disabilities among prisoners: Prevalence and mental and physical health comorbidities. *Journal of Applied Research in Intellectual Disabilities, 30*(2), 230–241.

Hussein, S., & Manthorpe, J. (2014). Structural marginalisation among the long-term care workforce in England: Evidence from mixed-effect models of national pay data. *Ageing and Society, 34*(1), 21–41.

Iacobucci, G. (2020). Covid-19: Racism may be linked to ethnic minorities' raised death risk, says PHE. *BMJ, 369*. https://doi.org/10.1136/bmj.m2421

Jegatheesan, B., Fowler, S., & Miller, P. J. (2010). From symptom recognition to services: How South Asian Muslim immigrant families navigate autism. *Disability and Society, 25*(7), 797–811.

Jenkins, R. (1998). *Questions of competence: Culture, classification and intellectual disability*. Cambridge: Cambridge University Press.

Johnson, M. (2008). Beyond *we care too*: Putting *Black carers in the picture*. London: Afiya Trust.

Jones, C. P. (2001). Invited commentary: 'Race,' racism, and the practice of epidemiology. *American Journal of Epidemiology, 154*(4), 299–304. https://doi.org/10.1093/aje/154.4.299

Keating, F., & Robertson, D. (2004). Fear, black people and mental illness: A vicious circle? *Health and Social Care in the Community, 12*(5), 439–447. https://doi.org/10.1111/j.1365-2524.2004.00506.x

Lintern, S. (2020). Hundreds of learning disability deaths in just eight weeks, new data show. *The Independent*, 19 May. www.independent.co.uk/news/health/coronavirus-learning-disability-nhs-england-mencap-a9522746.html

Malik, A., Boyle, B., & Mitchell, R. (2017). Contextual ambidexterity and innovation in healthcare in India: The role of HRM. *Personnel Review, 46*, 1358–1380. doi.org/10.1108/PR-06-2017-0194

Maylor, U. (2009). Is it because I'm Black? A Black female research experience. *Race Ethnicity and Education, 12*(1), 53–64. https://doi.org/10.1080/13613320802650949

Mehrotra, N., & Vaidya, S. (2008). Exploring constructs of intellectual disability and personhood in Haryana and Delhi. *Indian Journal of Gender Studies, 15*(2), 317–340. doi:10.1177/097152150801500206

Mir, G., Nocon, A., Ahmad, W., & Jones, L. (2001). *Learning disabilities and ethnicity*. London: Department of Health.

Moriarty, J. (2014). *Personalisation for people from black and minority ethnic groups*. London: Race Equality Foundation.

Netten, A., Jones, K., Knapp, M., Fernandez, J. L., Challis, D., Glendinning, C., Jacobs, S., Manthorpe, J., Moran, N., & Stevens, M. (2012). Personalisation through individual budgets: Does it work and for whom? *British Journal of Social Work, 42*(8), 1556–1573.

Newnes, C. (2018) The state and state(us) of clinical psychology. *Clinical Psychology Forum, 309*, 39–45.

O'Shaughnessy, D. F., & Tilki, M. (2007). Cultural competency in physiotherapy: A model for training. *Physiotherapy, 93*(1), 69–77. https://doi.org/10.1016/j.physio.2006.07.001

Parker, H. (1997). Beyond ethnic categories: Why racism should be a variable in health services research. *Journal of Health Services Research and Policy, 2*(4), 256–259. https://doi.org/10.1177/135581969700200411

Raghavan, R., & Waseem, F. (2007). Services for young people with learning disabilities and mental health needs from South Asian communities. *Advances in Mental Health and Learning Disabilities, 1*(3), 27–31.

Robertson, J., Raghavan, R., Emerson, E., Baines, S., & Hatton, C. (2019). What do we know about the health and health care of people with intellectual disabilities from minority ethnic groups in the United Kingdom? A systematic review. *Journal of Applied Research in Intellectual Disabilities, 32*(6), 1310–1334.

Saunders, A., Browne, D. & Durcan, D. (2013) *The Bradley Commission Briefing 1: Black and minority ethnic communities, mental health and criminal justice*. London: Centre for Mental Health.

Skills for Care. (2019). *The state of the adult social care sector and workforce in England*. London: Skills for Care Workforce Intelligence Team. www.skillsforcare.org.uk/stateof.

Stevens, M., Hussein, S., & Manthorpe, J. (2012). Experiences of racism and discrimination among migrant care workers in England: Findings from a mixed-methods research project. *Ethnic and Racial Studies, 35*(2), 259–280.

Talbot, J. (2008) *Prisoners' voices. Experiences of the criminal justice system by prisoners with learning disabilities and difficulties*. London: Prison Reform Trust.

Taylor, C. (2018). *Social care workforce study*. London: Care Association Alliance.

Trent Jr, J. W. (1994). *Inventing the feeble mind: A history of mental retardation in the United States* (vol. 6). Berkeley, CA: University of California Press.

Valuing People Support Team. (2004). *Green light for mental health*, parts A and B. London: Valuing People.

van Herwaarden, A., Rommes, E. W. M., & Peters-Scheffer, N. C. (2020). Providers' perspectives on factors complicating the culturally sensitive care of individuals with intellectual disabilities. *Research in Developmental Disabilities, 96*, 103543. https://doi.org/10.1016/j.ridd.2019.103543

Vertovec, S. (2007). Super-diversity and its implications. *Ethnic and Racial Studies, 30*(6), 1024–1054. DOI: 10.1080/01419870701599465

Webb, J., & Whitaker, S. (2012). Defining learning disability. *The Psychologist, 25*(6), 440–443.

Whyte, S. R. (1998). Slow cookers and madmen: Competence of heart and head in rural Uganda. *Questions of Competence: Culture, Classification and Intellectual Disability*, 153–175.

Williams, K., Papadopoulou, V., & Booth, N. (2012). *Prisoners' childhood and family backgrounds: Results from the Surveying Prisoner Crime Reduction (SPCR) longitudinal cohort study of prisioners*. London: Ministry of Justice. Available at: www.researchgate.net/profile/Natalie_Booth/publication/296701221_Prisoners'_Childhood_and_Family_Backgrounds/links/56d94afc08aee1aa5f817573.pdf.

Chapter 8

Judaism and the psy project

Craig Newnes

Summary

This chapter examines the Jewish origins of much of contemporary psy praxis and theory. It looks at founder figures in psychology and psychotherapy, the history of anti-semitism and violence linked to the psy project and recent examples of protestation, support and celebration of psy's Jewish heritage.

The roots of modernist psychology are a mixture of what now would be understood as racism, heterosexism and colonialism. These form the foundations of what kind of 'differences' might be explored and what kind of 'treatments' might be suggested for those seen as sufficiently beyond the arbitrary norms declared by a non-reflexive hegemony within the psy professions. Allied with notions of degeneration, the differences promoted by psy have led to othering, sterilisation and death-making (Wolfensberger, 1987). This chapter explores the roots of psychology in Judaism and the ways in which the psy project has both contributed to and resisted anti-semitism.

On being Jewish

Perhaps, it would be helpful to note that Judaism is, like many religions, not homogeneous. There are many different forms, for example, Reform, Conservative, Orthodox and Reconstructionist. Orthodox Judaism includes ultra-Orthodox (Haredi), Orthodox (including Hassidim), centrist Orthodox and Modern Orthodox. Others identify as 'nondenominational', 'trans-denominational', 'post-denominational' humanistic and the relatively recent, 'Jews for Jesus'.

There is a certain invisibility to being Jewish (Loewenthal, 2019; see Chapter 2, this volume). For example, despite for many years respecting Christian festivals the Division of Clinical Psychology (DCP) of the UK British Psychological Society (BPS) continued to arrange committee meetings at Rosh Hashanah or Yom Kippur. Even with a chairperson committed with her husband to observance committee meetings were timetabled on Jewish holidays.

I wasn't raised Jewish. My mum's mother had married out and, apart from the occasional Yiddish word got on with being what in the 16th century would have been known as a *converso* – not that she didn't act like a stereotypical Jewish matriarch. When her goy husband brought his mates round on shore leave during the Second World War her house became a (free) hotel for all and sundry. Did her generosity when I lived with her as a child influence my practice as a clinical psychologist and director of a psychological therapies department in a UK National Health Service Trust? I did my best to be available to staff, created a trust fund (from earnings as a lecturer and expert witness I was entitled to retain personally) that both provided a large departmental library and psychotherapy training for staff throughout the Trust, ensured service recipients were paid well for their role on interview panels long before other NHS departments followed suit, organised a staff counselling service and gave money to patients. No doubt the last would be regarded as a terrible breach of 'boundaries'. As Chair of the BPS Psychotherapy Section, perhaps I was leading the way; Freud believed in payment as part of the contract to the extent that he loaned money to the Wolf-man to pay for his analytic sessions – with Freud (Gardner, 1973).

Beyond that, my version of Judaism has elements of early Jewish thought. G-d is, quite literally, life. So we are all G-d, as are trees, breathing animals and the rest. Worshipping G-d is tricky and comes laden with all sorts of clutter – for Maimonides there are 613 mitzvot (duties). But worshipping life? What else is there? As a therapist I found suicide absurd. To kill all you have may be seen as understandable but, as Schopenhauer said, it illustrates that life is 'farce disguised as tragedy'. The threat of suicide brings out the worst in others. People who express the wish to die will be inscribed (diagnosed) with anything from depression to personality disorder and then subjected to well-meaning therapists offering moral orthopaedics, general practitioners prescribing psycho-active medication and psychiatrists suggesting electroshock (Newnes, 2018).

My mother's father had 18 brothers and sisters. The story was that three of his brothers went down on HMS *Hood* and his mum received three separate telegrams of condolence. One brother died in a straitjacket in Thorpe Asylum – my first introduction to psychiatry though, like the three naval brothers, his death was during World War II. I didn't come along until later.

By the time my grandad left to live – and eventually die – in a caravan in Fakenham alongside his lover I had another reason to fear psychiatry; in the 1950s and 1960s the usual warning in my neighbourhood to anyone who misbehaved was, 'You'll end up in Saint Nick's', the lunatic asylum on Great Yarmouth sea front. My beloved grandma spent two nights in that imposing place (see below).

Electroshock – called, for marketing purposes, Electro-Convulsive *Therapy* – was popular at Saint Nick's; electricity is a form of magic and psychiatry and psychology have a love affair with magic. Psy professionals target older women with electroshock. I loved my grandma; everyone did. Her father had the good sense to leave Germany at the end of the nineteenth century and eventually settled as a builder and undertaker. He was still alive when the synagogue in

Great Yarmouth was burned down in the 1920s – one reason that Jews became a serious minority on the East Anglian coast. My grandmother had distant cousins murdered in various camps during the Holocaust.

She eventually became – in her words – a bit 'doo-lally' and was found wandering around the garden by her neighbour who happened to be a social worker. She was admitted to Saint Nick's on a Friday; the day the hairdresser visited. Grandma's unkempt hair was unacceptable – so it was all shaved off. By Saturday she looked like any one of millions of faceless folk. But, for her, the transformation was like stepping back into a history of pogroms and worse.

During my career as a therapist, researcher, clinical psychologist and director of services I spent little time intending to hurt people. When patients said they felt better, I had no difficulty ending therapy and didn't chase patients who had come for only one session. As a manager I ensured that the majority of therapy staff in the department had individual and relatively private offices. The two psychotherapy centres had been modernised and provided free drinks and Internet access in comfortable waiting rooms; my version of being a good Jewish mother.

The history and nature of psy institutions might however suggest that my role was one of simply modernising the clinic – the Gaze and the essential power differentials between patients and 'experts' remained unaltered (Foucault, 1979). My stories to staff and patients about my bullied Jewish childhood and birth on a council estate can be seen as ploys to establish working-class (and oppressed) credentials amongst a group of predominantly working-class staff and patients. I was – sometimes – consciously using 'referent power' to gain influence[1] while the comfort of the waiting rooms can be seen as environments designed to seduce patients who, given the role of psychology and counselling in maintaining the status quo, should have maintained their wariness rather than submitting to the Gaze.

Judaism and psy

Some of the most basic facts collected at a psychological assessment session can highlight the difference between knowledge and knowing. With any luck clinicians in their sixties will record a date of birth pre-1953 with a different mind-set to a younger person. If a British resident, the clinician may have experienced rationing, some of the immediate after-effects of the Second World War (bomb craters and wrecked buildings following the Blitz were common in London until the 1960s), the years when young men were automatically recruited to the army and so on. Similarly, a Jewish clinician is likely to take more note of a new patient with the surname Levy or Cohen.

A list here of Jewish psy theorists and practitioners can barely do justice to the influence both Judaism and a rejection of Judaism has had within psy, and, by extension, the wider world. Adler, Bettleheim, Reik, Breuer, Rank, Klein and Erikson were, like Freud and of course his daughter Anna, all Jewish.

Alongside Freud, Sandor Ferenczi, Karl Abraham, Max Eitingon and Hans Sachs were all present at the first meeting of the International Psychoanalytical Congress, held in Salzburg in April 1908 after Ernest Jones had approached Jung the previous year (Davies, 1990). Jung eventually denounced Freudian psychoanalysis as a Jewish science unsuited to the Aryan soul (Karier, 1976).

Viktor Frankl was an Austrian neurologist and psychiatrist as well as a Holocaust survivor. Frankl was the founder of logotherapy, a form of existential analysis. His account of his life as a survivor and the foundations of logotherapy has been disputed, despite the sale of over 12,000,000 copies of *Man's Search for Meaning* (Frankl, 1959). The book chronicles Frankl's supposed experiences as a concentration camp inmate, which led him to discover the importance of finding meaning in all forms of existence, even the most brutal ones, and thus, a reason to continue living. It has been translated into 24 different languages. Frankl's mother Elsa and brother, Walter were murdered at Auschwitz. Frankl's wife was transported out of Auschwitz and moved to Bergen-Belsen where she too would be murdered.

Frankl has been the subject of criticism from several Holocaust analysts who questioned the levels of Nazi accommodation within the ideology of logotherapy and which Frankl personally willingly pursued in the time before his internment, when he voluntarily requested to perform unskilled lobotomy experiments approved by the Nazis on Jews (Pytell, 2003).

Man's Search for Meaning devotes almost half its contents to describing Auschwitz and the psychology of its prisoners, suggesting a long stay at the death camp. Frankl claimed to have survived Theresienstadt, Kaufering and Türkheim as well. His wording is, however, contradictory and to Pytell (2003), 'profoundly deceptive', as Frankl was held close to the train, in the 'depot prisoner' area of Auschwitz, for no more than a few days; he was neither registered there, nor assigned a number before being sent on to a subsidiary work camp of Dachau, known as Kaufering III, the true setting of much of what is described in his book.

In 1978 when attempting to give a lecture at the Institute of Adult Jewish Studies in New York, Frankl was confronted with an outburst of boos from the audience and was called a 'nazi pig' (Frankl#Controversy, 2019).

The founder of Gestalt therapy, Fritz Perls, was Jewish as were Albert Ellis (Rational Emotive Therapy), Arthur Janov (Primal therapy), Aaron Beck (Cognitive Behaviour Therapy) and Eric Berne (Transactional Analysis). Richard Bandler, co-creator of neuro-linguistic programming, and Francine Shapiro, creator of EMDR therapy, are Jewish.

In the world of academia Joseph Jastrow, whose father authored a Talmud dictionary, was the first recipient of an American Ph.D. in psychology in 1898 and established a psychological laboratory at the University of Wisconsin.

Psychological theorists including Asch, Festinger, Kohlberg, Lewin and Maslow were Jewish, as is Martin Seligman. Born in Poland in 1908, Else Frenkel-Brunswik was co-editor of the influential *The Authoritarian Personality.*

Like Freud, Erich Fromm, came from a family including several rabbis. The world's most used intelligence test and one integral to the training of UK clinical psychologists is named after its progenitor, David Wechsler. Another major influence on British clinical psychology in the 1960s was also Jewish, the South African psychiatrist, Joseph Wolpe. Monte Shapiro was also a South African Jewish émigré and first recipient of the British Psychological Society's award named in his honour in 1984.

There are critics as well as reactionaries amongst Jewish members of psy. Jewish psychiatrist and psychoanalyst Joseph Berke co-founded the Arbours Association in London having worked with renegade psychiatrist Ronnie Laing. David Rosenhan (Rosenhan, 1973) exposed the impoverishment of psychiatric diagnoses and George Weinberg coined the term 'homophobia'. Robert Jay Lifton and Erwin Staub have both written extensively on psy professionals' active involvement in genocide (Lifton, 1988; Staub, 1989). In contrast, John Glad's *Jewish Eugenics* (2011) controversially explores the Jewish history of ethnic cleansing of several millennia ago. The Torah, for example, includes G-d urging the Israelites to show no mercy towards the Hittites (Deuteronomy 7:3–4).

It would seem that the Jewish culture is integral to the psy project. An interpretation of the route to becoming a therapist that takes into account the influence of culture on beliefs and practices might note that the traditional role of rabbi/*rebbe* involves extensive counselling. Also: 'The *gabai* (rebbe's assistant) met with people before they met with the rebbe, and then: After interviewing the supplicant about his family, his background and his troubles, the gabai delivers the *kvitl* [written description of the presenting problem] and an oral report to the rebbe.' For some, this may resemble a typical psychotherapy or psychiatric intake session or assessment (Zborowski, & Herzog, 1995, 172).

Psychological and psychoanalytic theories also reflect the origins of their creators. For example, in Jewish tradition, the impulse to do good, the *yetzer hatov*, is balanced out by the *yetzer hara*, an inclination to destructiveness; a position that can be likened to Freud's notion of the life and death instincts (Kraft, n.d.).

A rejection of religious teaching had equally powerful effects on psy theorising. For example, although Freud would have been well aware of the Torah's proscription of sodomy as deserving of the death penalty (Leviticus 20:13), he positioned male homosexuality as a manifestation of *diverted* sexuality as an element of the Oedipus Complex (Freud, 1905/1962). He also acknowledged bisexuality as an innate disposition (Freud, 1926/1959).

'The first Lubavitcher Rebbe, Schneur Zalman … believed that the "animal soul", which has to do with physical pleasures, … and the "godly soul", which has to do with transcendent experience, were at war with each other' (Berke, 2015). The way to achieve at least momentary peace during this conflict is to physically experience transcendence through the touch and words of a loved one. Holding a loved child or true lover is thus transcendent. This form of transcendence may have led Perls to suggest sex with patients as curative, though less generous interpretations have been made.

A number of commentators and biographers have made direct links between Freudian theory and his Jewish heritage. Of equal importance to modern psy is the German philosophical tradition of the early 19th century. For example, Heinroth's *Lehrbuch der Störungen des Seelenlebens* (which Richards renders as Textbook of Disorders of the Soul) appeared in 1818. His system stresses madness having its source in sin and seems to predict Freud's tripartite division of the mind; the id, ego and superego are anticipated via the hedonistic/instinctual, central ego and conscience levels. The system uses an orthodox religious framework wherein submission to the demands of conscience lead to 'the sole path to God' (Richards, 1992, 314).

Heinroth (1993) also used a tripartite categorisation of mental disease; primary, secondary and transformed. The primary involved passion, delusion and vice residing in the heart, mind and will respectively. In secondary disease passion has developed into melancholy or senselessness, delusion into dullness or madness and vice into rage or shyness.

Dilemmas in psychology and psychotherapy of the 21st century – the importance of will, the centrality versus consequentiality of nature and nurture, the significance or otherwise of environment to unreason – much preoccupied German thinkers in the early 1800s. These debates formed the context for the rise in popularity of Freudian notions at the end of the century. Kant, for example, had suggested that the nature of the soul is rationally unknowable as – beyond the assertion, 'I think' – the essence of 'I' cannot be found. Although sensory experience is the basis for knowledge, processing of that experience follows *a priori* principles that do not themselves derive from experience – for example, time, space and causation. The world we experience – the phenomenal world – is constituted by our mind; the world as it is 'in itself' is beyond the grasp of reason. The mind's operations are here considered to be of three kinds: knowing, willing and feeling. These categories – again a tripartite system – were fundamental to later systems structuring the mind – for example, Freud's id, ego and superego; Berne's adult-parent-child; and the system of thought, behaviour and emotion central to Beck's Cognitive Behaviour Therapy (CBT). A recurring problem for psy is that any system of mind can only be theoretical. The idea, for example, that thoughts can influence feelings remains only an idea, despite its popularity with psy practitioners from CBT to dialectical behaviour therapy (DBT) via cognitive analytic therapists. There is an entire book to be written on the popularity of three letter acronyms in psy; virtually any combination of adjective (dynamic, cognitive, analytic, etc.) and further adjective or noun (family, individual, reality, etc.) can precede a therapy derivative (therapy, psychotherapy, analysis, etc.) to name a new intervention to add to the over 600 available. This number excludes many forms of indigenous ritual and moral orthopaedics practised for thousands of years (Feltham, 2013).

Anti-semitism

For all their influence on modernist psy praxis Judaism and Jews remain subject to anti-semitism, a 2,000-year history of exclusion and pogroms that reached their apogee in the years running up to and including the Holocaust.

In 19th-century France theories of the importance of hereditary were to the fore (Zola's Rougon-Macquart novels trace ongoing familial psychopathy back to Tante Dide in *La Bête Humaine*). A discourse in the 1860s on a Jewish propensity to mental illness (a trope used in later years by those fearing 'degeneration' in the Aryan and Anglo-Saxon gene pool) led to Charcot's treatment of 'Jewish nervous-ness' at the Saltpêtrière by the 1890s (Goldstein, 1985).

In early 19th-century Germany being Jewish was not regarded as a mental illness but was 'by definition a kind of criminality and immorality'. Ann Goldberg has examined the records of the Eberbach asylum in the duchy of Nassau, a territory bounded by Prussia to the north and west and Hesse-Darmstadt to the south and east. Nassau was notable for its range of represented religions including Lutherans, reformed Protestants, Catholics, Jews and Mennonites. To the extent that being Jewish was understood as a separate category with its own presumed hereditary and racial characteristics (principal amongst which was the notion of the *jüdischer Gauner* or Jewish crook) Jewish patients at the asylum avoided the medicalisation of conduct considered objectionable to the self or others. Jews in Nassau were denied civic rights and barred from certain trades and professions – an exclusion revisited in Germany in the 1920s. As a relatively poor group, their incarceration reflected pauperisation and the effects of living in a hostile environment. Despite these obvious factors any anti-social behaviour and associated 'criminality' were seen as an element of a *jüdischer Gauner* character rather than mental illness (Goldberg, 1999).

In 1899 the industrialist and social Darwinist Friedrich Kruup funded the Jena prize for a scientific answer to the question, 'What can we learn from the principles of evolution for the development of laws and states?' The closing date was 1 December 1902. The winning entrant, Shallmayer, used Weismann's theories of selectionist biology to formulate a code of 'generative ethics' – the 'unfit' would be prevented from reproducing. The degenerative included 'the insane, the feeble-minded, the alcoholic, those infected by TB and VD, and criminals' (Weindling, 1989).

Over the following years the theories of Hegar and of Shallmayer became part of the justificatory rhetoric for forced sterilisation in many industrialised countries including the US and Germany. In the late 1930s the theory of degeneration with its blend of biology and implications for state welfare and economic health allowed murder to take place in psychiatric hospitals in Germany.

Hitler's first declarations against the weak, whose lives were 'burdensome' for the state had been at the Nuremberg Party rally of 1929. After he gained power there was a relentless progression to the 'final solution' in which psychiatry would be a forerunner:

> While 'euthanasia' of the supposedly incurable was supported and legitimised by Hitler … medical experts took a crucial role in its administration … The victims were primarily children of under three years of age, diagnosed as mentally retarded or congenitally malformed, and the mentally ill.
>
> (Lifton, 1988)

A group including Phillippe Bouhler, Victor Brack (Hitler's physician) and the paediatricians Wentzler and Catel initiated killing under the auspices of the 'Reich Committee for the Scientific Registration of Serious Hereditary and Congenital Illnesses.'

In October 1939 Hitler enabled Bouhler and Brandt to begin *Gnatentod* (mercy killing) of patients judged incurable. The psychiatric team responsible for implementing *Gnatentod* was soon joined by an advocate of insulin shock, Nitsche. In December 1939 Jewish and Polish patients from Meseritz-Obrawalde were killed by a strong sedative (in woods nearby the hospital). Staff tried gassing patients as a more efficient method of killing and in June 1940 the gassing of Jewish patients began.

The first gas chambers were constructed in German hospitals. The aim was to kill via carbon monoxide or starvation patients incarcerated and inscribed as psychotic and children said to have genetic illnesses. In 1941 Eugen Fischer (who lived on for over 20 years after the war), the co-director of the Kaiser Wilhelm Institute for Archaeology, declared Bolsheviks and Jews to be a distinct degenerative species. And once an entire race is no longer considered human, the way is opened up for members to be herded up and slaughtered (Newnes, 2018).

Frank Zappa's ability to outrage anyone at all in the name of free speech was legendary – Jewish Princess from *Sheikh Yerbouti* includes the line, 'she's got a garlic aroma that could level Tacoma'. Within the tribe anti-semitic jokes are sometimes, just about, acceptable (Lenny Bruce and Woody Allen are but two in a long-line of comedians more qualified than most to get laughs for in-jokes). In an age where anti-semitism and conspiracy theories are on the rise, Zappa's line would no longer be tolerated.

As one example, Jew Watch promotes Holocaust denial and allegations of a conspiracy that Jews control the media and banking. There are also accusations of Jewish involvement in terrorist groups. If one's view is that one person's terrorist is another's freedom fighter, then MOSSAD might fall into either category, although the website presents neither a subtle reading – nor evidence (Jew Watch, 2020).

The conflation of Judaism with criminality (see above) is continued in numerous anti-semitic websites; one accuses Marx of being a 'Jewish parasite, liar, ideology warrior posing as an economist', and Einstein of being a 'Jewish parasite, liar, possible paedophile, ideology warrior posing as physicist', adding that Freud was a 'Jewish parasite, liar, ideology warrior posing as "psychologist"'. Freud was a neurologist before founding psychoanalysis. There are two psychologists on the site: David Wechsler, who again is presented as a 'Jewish parasite, liar, ideology warrior posing as "psychologist"' and B. F. Skinner (who was an avowed atheist), positioned as a 'Jewish parasite, psychopath posing as psychologist (the lunatics are running the asylum).' The inaccuracy and venom is compounded by misspelling posing as 'possing' throughout (metadave, 2020).

Love ...

Students of irony might appreciate that even Carl Rogers' – himself born into an 'almost fundamentalist Christian family' (Feltham, 2013) – most well-known factor in successful psychotherapy – unconditional positive regard – is, ultimately derived from the Jewish sage Hillel (c.110 BCE–10 CE). When asked to recite the Torah while standing on one leg the rabbi offered the golden rule: 'That which is hateful to you, do not do to your fellow. That is the whole Torah; the rest is the explanation; go and learn.' Sometimes this is presented as 'Love a stranger as we would ourselves – the rest is commentary.' It would seem a good place to start.

Note

1 This paragraph first appeared in Newnes, 2016, 161. French and Raven (1959), in examining social power, found referent power (i.e., the perception that the other person is essentially similar to you in status or culture) as the most influential. Undeniably, reward power and the legitimate power of authority are vested in the consultant's ability to discharge the patient, but in day-to-day life on the wards referent power is key.

References

Berke, J. H. (2015). *The hidden Freud: His Hassidic roots*. London: Karnac Book.

Davies, T. G. (1990). 'Truth is a point of view.' An account of the life of Dr. Ernest Jones. In R. M. Murray and T. H. Turner (Eds.). *Lectures on the history of psychiatry: The Squibb series*. London: Gaskell/Royal College of Psychiatrists.

Feltham, C. (2013). *Counselling and counselling psychology: A critical examination*. Ross-on-Wye: PCCS Books.

Foucault, M. (1979). *Discipline and punish*. Harmondsworth: Penguin.

Frankl, V. (1959). *Man's search for meaning: An introduction to logotherapy*. New York: Touchstone.

Frankl#Controversy (2019). https://en.wikipedia.org/wiki/Viktor_Frankl#Controversy. Accessed 8 May 2019.

French, J. R. P., & Raven, B. (1959). The bases of social power. In D. Cartwright & A. Zander (Eds.). Group dynamics (pp. 150–167). New York: Harper & Row.

Freud, S. (1905/1962). *Three essays on the theory of sexuality*. Drei Abhandlungen zur Sexualtheorie. Trans. J. Strachey. New York: Basic Books.

Freud, S. (1926/1959). *The question of lay analysis.* Trans. J. Strachey in the Standard Edition. London: Hogarth Press and the Institute of Psycho-Analysis.

Gardner, M. (Ed.) (1973). *The wolf-man and Sigmund Freud.* London: Hogarth Press.

Glad, J. (2011). *Jewish eugenics.* Washington, DC: Wooden Shore Publishers. www.woodenshore.org.

Goldberg, A. (1999). *Sex, religion and the making of modern madness: The Eberbach asylum and German society 1815–1849.* Oxford: Oxford University Press.

Goldstein, J. (1985). The wandering Jew and the problem of psychiatric anti-Semitism in fin-de-siècle France. *Journal of Contemporary History, 20,* 521–552. https://doi.org/10.1177/002200948502000403

Heinroth, J. C. A. (1993). L. A re-examination. In L. de Goei and J. Vijselaar (Eds.). *Proceedings: 1st European Congress on the History of Mental Health Care* (pp. 8–12). Rotterdam: Erasmus Publishing.

Jew Watch (2020). https://en.wikipedia.org/wiki/Jew_Watch. Accessed. 9 May 2019.

Karier, C. (1976). The ethics of a therapeutic man. In G. Kren & L. Rappoport (Eds.). *Varieties of psychohistory* (pp. 333–363). New York: Springer.

Kraft, J. (n.d.). *Judaism and psychology.* www.myjewishlearning.com/article/judaism-and-psychology/ Accessed 8 May 2019.

Lifton, R. J. (1988). *The Nazi doctors: Medical killing and the psychology of genocide.* London: Little Brown Book Group.

Loewenthal, K. (2019). Invisible anti-semitism in clinical psychology. Presentation at the Invisible Racism symposium. Division of Clinical Psychology Annual Conference, 24 January, Salford, UK.

metadave (2020). https://metadave.wordpress.com/2007/06/25/jewish-a-priori-junk-science/ Accessed 9 May 2019.

Newnes, C. (2016). *Clinical psychology: A critical examination.* Monmouth: PCCS Books.

Newnes, C. (2018). Death-making and David Reville. In *A critical A-Z of electroshock* (pp. 36–46). London: Real Press.

Pytell, T. E. (2003). Redeeming the unredeemable: Auschwitz and man's search for meaning. Holocaust and Genocide Studies, *17*(1), 89–113. Project MUSE muse.jhu.edu/article/43137

Richards, G. (1992). *Mental machinery,* Part 1, *The origins and consequences of psychological ideas 1600–1850.* London: Athlone Press.

Rosenhan, D. L. (1973). On being sane in insane places. *Science, 179*(4070), 250–258. DOI: 10.1126/science.179.4070.250

Staub, E. (1989). *The roots of evil: The origins of genocide and other group violence.* New York: Cambridge University Press.

Weindling, P. (1989). *Health, race and German politics between national unification and Nazism 1870–1945.* Cambridge: Cambridge University Press.

Wolfensberger, W. (1987). *The new genocide of handicapped and afflicted people.* New York: University of Syracuse.

Zborowski, M., and Herzog, E. (1995). *Life is with people: The culture of the shtetl.* New York: Schocken Books.

Chapter 9

Racism in New Zealand psychology, or, would Western psychology be a good thing?

Pikihuia Pomare, Julia Ioane, and Keith Tudor

Summary

This chapter offers critical reflections on the influence and institutions of psychology in Aotearoa New Zealand. While we generally consider that psychology encompasses the psy disciplines, i.e. counselling, psychology, and psychotherapy, in this chapter and given our respective professional backgrounds and identities, we focus more on clinical psychology and psychotherapy. Weaving together our own stories of place, space, and belonging, the chapter discusses our different experiences of how some of the assumptions implicit in Western psychology impact on the education/training and culture of the psy professions and complex, as well as their clinical practice, and the resistance to changing this. Written and edited together, while also acknowledging our individual experiences and voices, the chapter addresses the question of how a critique based on a decolonising perspective could lead to a psychology that serves the health and well-being of all the people of Aotearoa New Zealand.

> Tūngia te ururua kia tupu whakaritorito te tupu o te harakeke | Clear the undergrowth so the new shoots of the flax will grow.
>
> British Journalist: What do you think of Western civilisation?
> Mahatma Gandhi: I think it would be a good idea.

Whiri | Strands

Pikihuia: I was born in Hokianga, Northland, and lived in a small rural community in the south side of the Hokianga called Koutu, not far from Opononi, well-known for its picturesque harbour views, sand dunes and Opo, the friendly dolphin who visited there in the 1950s. Hokianga is a community that is well known for having an eclectic mix of people: hippies from all over the world and around Aotearoa New Zealand who lived off the land, comparatively well-off Pākehā (NZ European) farmers and local Māori (Indigenous New Zealanders) also referred to as tāngata whenua (first peoples/people of the land) from local hapū (sub-tribe(s)) and iwi (tribe(s)) who had lived there since the tūpuna (ancestors) from Polynesia arrived in Aotearoa New Zealand between 1,000 and 2,000 years ago (Howe, 2006). I remember attending lots of hui (meetings/gatherings) throughout Northland. We were the first generation to attend Kōhanga Reo (Māori immersion pre-school) as a result of activism groups like Ngā Tama Toa that my parents were members of. Although we were surrounded by different groups of people, for me, being Māori was the norm. At 6 years of age, we moved to Auckland and my mother told me a story of how she took us to Queen Street, the main street in Auckland City. When I got off the bus, I looked up the road and, upon seeing all the people, said to her, 'Do I have to hongi all these people, mum?' (A hongi is a unique Māori greeting that was part of my everyday social way of interacting with others.) That was what we did – and still do – in the Hokianga. We had moved to Auckland so my mother could retrain as a teacher and so we went to a Kura Kaupapa Māori (Māori immersion school), one of the first in Aotearoa New Zealand.

Kura Kaupapa Māori were established in the late 1980s with the explicit intent to provide a Māori environment to educate Māori children in te reo Māori (the Māori language), we learnt all of subjects in Māori and were imbued with Māori philosophies and protocols that enabled us not only to be successful but also to stand strong as Māori in the world. Later, I came to learn that what we were being taught came from Māori epistemologies, also known in Aotearoa as Mātauranga Māori. Our Indigenous worldview was taken as matter of fact and the focus was on both our academic and our spiritual development in order to fulfil our potential. Te Aho Matua, the guiding philosophy of Kura Kaupapa Māori, starts with a whakataukī (proverb) that states: 'He kākano ahau i rūia mai i Rangiātea, e kore ahau e ngaro' (I will never be lost for I am a seed that was sown in Rangiātea), thereby emphasising our past and present collective connection and reinforcing our belonging and identity. The fact that we spoke Māori, despite the efforts of colonisation to eradicate our language with the Native Schools Act (in place from 1888 to 1969), was an act of reasserting our rangatiratanga (authority/self-determination). Generations who came before me – my father, my grandparents, and their parents – all attended 'Native Schools'. The aim was to assimilate Māori children into Pākehā society because being Māori and speaking Māori was considered inferior, a common narrative as part of the colonial conditioning of the mind, 'being and speaking Māori does not get you anywhere'. Māori children were disciplined and physically punished for speaking Māori at school. Both the physical and the psychological trauma that children experienced at the hands of teachers who were agents of the Crown (the New Zealand State) is still felt today. I had an insight into the attitudes of general society towards Māori through interactions we had; for example, we were told (by both Pākeha and Māori) that we would not succeed in education because we went to Kura (Māori immersion school). Sports were seen as another area for failure; I recall one year our Kura team was in the A grade for netball in central Auckland and another team from an affluent suburb made an official complaint about us speaking Māori to each other on the court. Although this happened in the 1990s, I have heard of similar stories and incidents in more recent years.

I am acutely aware of the privilege I hold of being able to speak my reo freely while many of my kin, whānau (extended family) and previous generations before me did not have the option of being raised in Māori immersion environments; they were not provided the space in an education system that encouraged them to privilege their whakapapa (genealogy) and identity. Rather, generations of Māori experienced racist attitudes of teachers: being told that they were less capable than their Pākehā contemporaries and being explicitly encouraged to pursue low-paying jobs. This has had significant psychological and economic impacts for generations of Māori. In order for me to receive any of the rights and benefits to my own language and our knowledge systems by way of Kōhanga Reo and Kura Kaupapa Māori, Māori activists had to apply significant pressure via resistance movements against the Crown to recognise Māori rights under Te Tiriti o Waitangi (the Treaty of Waitangi), the founding document of this nation, signed in 1840 by Māori Rangatira (chiefs) and representatives of the British Crown, which, amongst other things, promised a joint Māori–Crown relationship (see Treaty2U, 2020).

Given this background, my initial experiences of becoming immersed in the Pākehā world came as a cultural shock, though at the time my understanding was that this was just how things were. After my primary schooling in Kura Kaupapa I went to Pākehā schools (also known as mainstream schools) and then to university to study psychology. At the high school I attended I met other Māori who had internalised racist and deficit stereotypes about being Māori. One of the most harmful ways in which colonisation continues to infect us is the colonisation of the mind, our Māori psyche, brainwashing us to believe that we are somehow an inferior race.

Studying psychology, I found it interesting learning about people and how they thought. Social psychology and clinical psychology interested me because of my upbringing and being raised politically and socially conscious from a young age. What became apparent, however, was that Indigenous Māori perspectives on and of psychology rarely featured in our curriculum. I counted four individual lectures in my entire undergraduate degree that had a Māori focus, with a handful in my clinical psychology training delivered by dedicated Māori staff who were often expected to make up for the entire system that privileged Pākehā knowledge. This was a stark contrast to the depth of Mātauranga (knowledge) in which I had been immersed, and which clearly demonstrated the existence of an Indigenous psychology here in Aotearoa New Zealand. Yet the theories and practices from psychology that were being applied to Māori in child protection, education, forensic, justice, mental health and other sectors was imported from North America and Europe and, specifically, the United Kingdom. There were several standout experiences of racism from my peers during my clinical training, including the refusal of some to attend a marae (cultural meeting house) for cultural competency training.

Some of reasons given for not wanting to stay at the marae exemplify the racist rhetoric that existed then and persists now.

Julia: As a child of the Pasifika diaspora, growing up in South Auckland (where the majority of Pasifika communities in this country live) was filled with many happy memories and adventures. (The word and term Pasifika includes someone born in or a descendent of those born in the Pacific Islands, and includes Polynesia, Melanesia and Micronesia in the South Pacific.) As I reflect on my childhood as an adult, I recall the moments of racism and discrimination, though as a child, these were normal. I accepted it because I was raised to understand the sacrifices my parents had made in their migration to Aotearoa New Zealand. Reciprocity to parents is a key value of being Pasifika (Ioane, 2017), which, for me, was to benefit from a good education and do better than the life in which I was raised. That took priority; everything else, including racism and discriminatory remarks made by others towards me, was simply ignored. In addition, there was a safe and supportive network in South Auckland where most people looked like me and so I didn't really need to think about the 'other'. Going to university was pretty much the same as you stuck to the same circle of friends and network – people that looked like you. My parents also encouraged us to hang out with pālagi friends (Pālagi is the Samoan term for European or Pākehā people), so we could learn their ways of living and try to adapt, though it was clear that this was only for outside the family home and to get ahead in life.

Looking back, my training as a psychologist was extremely limited in terms of Pasifika worldviews and ways of knowing. It is important, however, to remember that I came from an era of first-generation NZ-born Samoans where our main goal was to get educated and contribute to the family. Culture and family was strong, with those principles taught within the family home. There was no expectation that I would find my Pacific identity in education or employment as home provided my identity in abundance. That was my upbringing. I enjoyed my training in psychology, though I can understand now why many would not see it in the same way. As cultures evolve, and communities increase in diversity, the need for psychology to reflect the society that we live in remains (Theule & Germain, 2017).

When I became a psychologist, further moments of racism and discrimination come to mind. In my work in Youth Justice, I was often mistaken for the mother or relative of a young person, usually of Māori or Pasifika descent. Professionally, I was assumed to be the youth worker or social worker (both professions have large numbers of Pasifika). To date, I have never had anyone (Pacific or non-Pacific) correctly identify me as a psychologist in a first meeting. Despite these moments, I am in a privileged position with an opportunity to advocate for our Indigenous and ethnic minorities as I sit at the same table as colleagues from dominant and Western worldviews. Many times, I am the only brown face in a sea of white: I look different and my opinions are different. During my early career, my voice was hardly shared, however over time I have learnt to challenge respectfully.

My most recent and perhaps most stand-out 'racist' moments for me come from my work in academia. When I arrived, most colleagues assumed that I must be studying for my doctorate (I already had one); one colleague, with whom I'd sat in team meetings for more than a year, told me quite bluntly that I was not a clinical psychologist (I had been – for almost ten years). According to others, I only got (into) these positions or roles because I was Pasifika or because others were Māori. Very few want to hear about the injustices we may have experienced or the numerous times in which we have been overlooked or shut down because we do not represent or express the dominant Western worldview. To some people in the field of psychology (practice, profession and discipline), I am where I am because of my ethnicity and being Pasifika is my expertise. Not so. Pasifika is my identity *and* expertise, though it is *not* my only expertise.

I am contributing to this chapter because I have first-hand personal and professional experiences of the racism that continues to exist in psychology and the other psy disciplines. First, I have seen this in the recruitment of students to psychology; second, in the curriculum; third, among colleagues and the culture of psychology itself. In my view, it is challenging to accept/acknowledge other worldviews, particularly when they are so different from your own. Non-Pasifika communities continue to tell us as Pasifika what we need to know and how we should respond and resolve the issues in our communities. Whilst we have been asked what we think, the implementation of what we think is where the challenge lies. I recently had a student ask me how we could work effectively with Pasifika. My response was 'Ask them.' Whilst this may sound simple, it requires you as the (dominant) 'other' to acknowledge that you don't know the answer, and, perhaps more importantly, that you have to share power. Both of these (not knowing and power sharing) remain a challenge both in psychology and society at large.

Keith: In 2008, I came to New Zealand primarily to attend the New Zealand Association of Psychotherapists' annual conference which, that year, was held at Waitangi, both at Te Tii marae and the Copthorne Hotel, Waitangi (though, interestingly and, I think, significantly, its advertised address is 'Bay of Islands'), venues that, in themselves, were and are a symbolic representation of ngā ao e rua, the (meeting of the) two worlds in Aotearoa New Zealand, that is Māori and non Māori. Indeed, a significant element of what was an exceptionally well-planned and inspiring conference was the daily walk across the bridge between the two venues. As a participant in the conference, I also had the privilege of being welcomed onto the marae and was one of about 50 people who chose to stay overnight in the whare nui (the big meeting house) for the duration of the conference. At the conference, I remember one particularly inspiring presentation, by Bronwyn Campbell, a Māori psychologist, at the beginning of which she spoke some te reo (Māori). I was sitting next to two older colleagues in the psychotherapy community, one of whom, after a while, whispered to the other: 'Why do they have to talk so much Māori?'

I was shocked on a number of levels and for a number of reasons, which, here, I describe, and link to the broader issue of racism in psychology and, in this case, psychotherapy.

First, with regard to language – te reo is both the first language and an official language of New Zealand. Since the initiatives to revitalise the language in the 1970s, it has increasingly been used by Māori and non Māori as part of welcoming, acknowledging and introducing people in formal and relatively informal occasions such as a presentation. At the time, I didn't understand any te reo but, at that particular moment (in the seminar), I enjoyed hearing the language. I was raised in the UK with a love of languages. My father was a teacher of German language and literature. We often had German students staying with us; and, when we went abroad on family holidays, my parents encouraged my brothers and me to learn some of the basics expressions of the language of the country in which we were staying. Later, in my early thirties, I lived in Italy for two years and learned Italian, as part of which I have many experiences, both comfortable and uncomfortable, of sitting in groups (in social occasions, classes and at small and large events) not understanding very much of what was being said. However, in some way, I was learning to listen beyond or underneath the content and explicit language being used (for a model about which, see Fleming, 1984). I appreciate that these particular personal experiences have given me a greater tolerance for not understanding as part of a process of learning. Nevertheless, I suggest that, and especially from a psychological point of view, it is important to be and to remain open to experience (Rogers, 1959), and, in this context, for Pākehā and Tau Iwi (new incomers) to be open to listening to the experience of Māori in their own land. With regard to psychology and working therapeutically, I link this to the concepts of contact (Rogers, 1957; 1959) and clinical hospitality (Orange, 2012). As a relative newcomer (I emigrated here with my family in 2009), it seems to me a simple matter of common courtesy to be able to greet people in the first language of the country, and, preferably, to be able to observe and engage in the basic rituals of contact, welcome, engagement, dialogue and hospitality. Fortunately, I am not alone in thinking along these lines. Earlier this year, the New Zealand government passed the Health Practitioners Competence Assurance Amendment Act 2020, which amongst other things amended the previous version of the Act with regard to cultural competence as follows: 'In section 118(i), replace "cultural competence" with "cultural competence (including competencies that will enable effective and respectful interaction with Māori)"' (Section 37(2)).

Second, with regard to the use of the word 'they' – in the original incident, the colleague's use of the word 'they' was delivered with a certain disdain, which, along with the fact that she used the plural, seemed to reflect a generalised ('they', referring to all Māori) as well as a distal (us and them) relationship between the colleague and the presenter. Many psy practitioners will be familiar with the psychoanalytic concept of 'the other' and 'othering', by which the person or persons other than the subject is/are viewed as the object of projection(s): as strange, foreign, dangerous, exotic, etc., and demonised or idealised, but, in any case, marginalised. Of course, this is especially poignant when, as a result of colonisation, including disease and deaths, and the non-Māori population surpassing the Indigenous Māori population within less than 20 years of the first settlements, it is Māori who become the 'other' in their own country. One of the effects of this is to maintain the dominant subject as central and supposedly neutral. In her book, *Southern theory*, Cornell (2008) critiques the notion of the Western – and Northern – intellectual tradition being central, arguing that 'colonised and peripheral societies produce social thought about the modern world which has as much intellectual power as metropolitan social thought, and more political relevance' (p. xii). Elsewhere, I have applied this critique to psychotherapy and offered a view of 'Southern psychotherapies' (Tudor, 2012). In the same vein, I would argue that we need to challenge the assumption of neutrality in psychology and the psy professions.

There was a third aspect to this incident which was the context, that is, the subject of Bronwyn Campbell's talk, which began with some history and some challenges to traditional views of New Zealand history, which were illustrated with reference to a number of different flags (see Tudor, 2016).

Is New Zealand racist?

New Zealand has a reputation not only for being beautiful, clean and green, but for having good race relations. This myth was both represented and challenged in an interview by Alex Denny of *Dazed and Confused*, with Unknown Mortal Orchestra's Ruban Nielsen and New Zealand filmmaker Taika Waititi in 2018:

ALEX DENNY: I think I've got quite an idealised vision of New Zealand as like Australia without the racism and the blokeish sense of humour …

TAIKA WAITITI: Nah, it's racist as fuck. I mean, I think New Zealand is the best place on the planet, but it's a racist place. People just flat-out refuse to pronounce Māori names properly. There's still profiling when it comes to Polynesians. It's not even a colour thing – like, 'Oh, there's a black person.' It's, 'If you're Poly then you're getting profiled.'

RUBAN NIELSON: I didn't even realise how light my skin was until I came (to the US). It was one of the things I liked when I moved here; it's like nobody knows what you are so they give you the benefit of the doubt. And then I go back to New Zealand as a person who's older and somewhat accomplished in their field and I still get treated worse! It's like people want to remind you – 'Yeah, but you're still Polynesian, so …'

TAIKA WAITITI: Totally. People in Auckland are very patronising. They're like, 'Oh, you've done so well, haven't you? For how you grew up. For one of your people.'

Part of the reason that we quote this here is because, given Taika Waititi's high profile in the country, it led to some backlash and quite a debate about racism in New Zealand.

Julia: Taika and Ruban are spot on with their commentary. From my experience, those of us who agree with their views have and have had direct experience or exposure to these general stereotypes of who we are. One that quickly springs to mind was when I was talking to a senior academic and manager in psychology who said to me 'Gosh, there aren't many people like you in our field, you must be so happy … So, do Tongans and Samoans speak the same language?' Another (more) junior psychologist was introduced to me and told that I teach in the university; her response was: 'Congratulations that you're in the programme; all the best with your studies.' Those who didn't agree with the comments made by Taika and Ruban appear to come from non Māori/Pasifika/ethnic minority communities with no awareness of the diversity within these communities, nor the histories of colonisation that have impacted our development in Aotearoa New Zealand. Furthermore, it is difficult to see the gaps when you live in an environment that promotes choice and equality without first looking at the privilege one lives within.

Keith: For my part, as a white man, I haven't experienced racism (though I have experienced quite strong anti-British sentiment in New Zealand), but I have certainly witnessed racism, as well as strong resistance to anti-racist and progressive policies, procedures and practice. One of my earliest experiences since emigrating here in 2009 was with a colleague in psychology who responded to my advocay of biculturalism and honouring Te Tiriti o Waitangi (in line with the University's Directions), by advising me against, as he put it, 'getting down with the Brown'. I challenged him about this language and, although he obviously felt no compunction in expressing his view in this way, judging by his reaction to my challenge, he was less open to hearing my view; and we have barely talked in the ten years since.

Pikihuia: My question is whether psychology itself is another form of colonisation? When we look at the history of psychology in this country, it has come from Western academic scientific psychology; its knowledge and research is based primarily on Western educated industrialised rich democratic countries/populations that comprise 12% of the world's population (Berry et al., 2002). The whakapapa of psychology as a discipline needs to be acknowledged in the context of racism and power because of how knowledge in the discipline is valued and positioned. In my profession of clinical psychology, knowledge is often compartmentalised, for example, Western theories, models, paradigms and professional practice are positioned as 'clinical', while Māori knowledge and practices are 'cultural'. Clinical knowledge is often used as a way of communicating which is precise, accurate, evidence-based and safe. In contrast, cultural knowledge and competencies are often perceived as an adjunct and complementary to the 'real' work. In the psy professions, there are racial hierarchies of what is valued and considered valid. That is not to say that Western knowledge has no utility for Māori but, rather, that it is not offered the same status or space to understand and work with Māori in practice. Māori knowledge appears to be to an afterthought, if acknowledged at all. The suppression of Māori cosmologies, ontologies, epistemologies and methodologies through colonisation has had a huge impact on Māori well-being, as is evident in the high burden of distress brought about by a myriad of factors that have resulted in economic disadvantage/deprivation and social harms. For example, the Tohunga Suppression Act 1907 (which was only repealed in 1962) severed Māori knowledge transmission about health (for a discussion; see Woodard, 2014). Likewise, the confiscation of whenua (land) impacted on Māori not only economically but also dislocated Māori from health practices that were based on an intimate and symbiotic relationship with the natural environment. Māori have disproportionately high rates of suicide (Ministry of Health, 2016). Māori rates of imprisonment are also disproportionate and stand at 50% for Māori males and 60% for Māori females (Māori comprise 16.5% of the general population: Statistics New Zealand, 2019). There are also disproportionately high rates of removal of Māori children by the state (Office of the Children's Commissioner, 2020); of ill-health and psychiatric diagnoses amongst Māori and of compulsory treatment orders (Elder & Tapsell, 2013); and of seclusion and restraint (Wharewera-Mika et al., 2016). What we are grappling with here is a humanitarian crisis in our own country, created by ongoing colonisation and fostered and still fuelled by racism.

We give these examples to assert, alongside Taika Waititi, Ruban Nielsen and many others, that New Zealand is racist but that, given its history since its colonisation, this is hardly surprising. The point is to acknowledge it and to change. In this, we think that psychologists and therapists have a key role as we know that awareness and motivation come before change. Thus, acknowledgement of the reality of racism comes before anti-racist praxis; and acknowledgement of New Zealand's history, including British colonisation, is a prerequisite of decolonisation.

The point is to change it

To paraphrase Karl Marx (1888/1972) (who was referring to philosophers), we would say that most of the psychologists and psychotherapists have only *interpreted* the world, in various ways; 'the point, however, is to *change* it' (p. 13). There are, of course, honourable exceptions, including various traditions of radical therapy (for a critical review and overview of which, see Tudor & Begg, 2016). The US radical psychiatrists, for example, argued that 'Therapy is change, not adjustment. [and that] This *means* change – social, personal, and political.' (Anon., 1973, p. xi).

Tūngia te ururua kia tupu whakaritorito te tupu o te harakeke. In the spirit of this whakataukī, we conclude this chapter by making some suggestions as to what undergrowth needs to be cleared in order for the new shoots of the flax to grow.

Decolonising the curriculum

Although students and academics have been talking about decolonising curricula for a number of years, this gained momentum following protests initiated by South African university students under the banners of #RhodesMustFall, #Fees Must Fall – and, indeed, the statue of Sir Cecil John Rhodes was removed from the University of Cape Town in April 2015. While the debate about decolonising the curriculum ensues, relatively little has changed. Following the protest, and listening to students, Shay (2016), a South African academic, identified a number of challenges which, she argued could and should form a strategy for such decolonisation, i.e., #1 that the curriculum needs to be fit for purpose, and #2 relevant to the real world; #3 that, in any redesign of the curriculum, student voices must be heard; #4 that a decolonised curriculum needs to challenge the dominant worldview (and represent different worldviews), as well as #5 power plays by academics who are either abusive or unaware of their power and privilege; and #6 that all aspects of the curriculum (and the systems that support it) need to change in order to challenge and change inequalities. We agree with Shay's points and see the need for this kind of strategy here in Aoteroa New Zealand.

In response to these points, we consider (with regard to #1 and #2) that, with few exceptions, the curricula of education/training in the psy professions in tertiary institutions in the country are neither fit for purpose nor relevant to our current or future real world. Reviews of professional psychology training programmes at universities in Aotearoa New Zealand found substantial issues with the teaching of Māori content with regard to knowledge, skills, practice and cultural competence (Levy & Waitoki, 2015). As these inadequacies place a significant barrier for Māori students, decolonising and Indigenising the curriculum and the pedagogy would not only be 'a good thing' but would and should also be a major incentive for attracting and retaining Māori in the profession. When we look at the curricula of the psy disciplines across the board, there is, and with a few notable exceptions, little recognition or knowledge of Indigenous and Pasifika worldviews theory or practice (Ioane & Lambie, 2016). For example, the Western theory of human attachment implies one primary (maternal) caregiver, whereas, among more collective communities and collectivist cultures, there are usually multiple carers to which the child has multiple attachments (Mikahere-Hall, 2020). In terms of how the external world impacts on the curriculum, in this country a review of any curriculum will immediately reveal whether and to what extent:

1. It is informed by and applying the Articles of Te Tiriti o Waitangi.
2. It is teaching and examining Pasifika and other worldviews in psychology.
3. The staff is competent in doing the above (in terms of ontologies, epistemologies, methodologies, and method/practice) and in sharing the curriculum and teaching space with other worldviews.

We would suggest that such a review would reveal that most curricula in the education/training in the psy professions would not pass these criteria/tests and, therefore, that much needs to be done. In our experience and, given the dominance of Western educated/trained Pākehā academics, it appears challenging to many of them to integrate Māori and Pasifika worldviews, perhaps because it highlights the inadequacies in their own worldviews to acknowledge and address indigeneity.

Keith: One of my early experiences as a member of a faculty board of studies, was seeing a number of instances in which academics were proposing to delete references to the Treaty of Waitangi (the founding document of our nation) in order to make the paper (course) or programme more appealing to a wider (and international) audience. Fortunately, with the support of another senior colleague, we were able to resist and challenge this, and:

a. to have the discussion about the uniqueness of our cultural context in this country, and that this is important, not least to international students;
b. to reassert the importance of honouring the Treaty, and as part of which of referring to it as Te Tiriti o Waitangi, with the important implication that we are honouring the Māori version of it; and
c. in the context of the particular faculty, to link the inclusion of Te Tiriti in the curriculum to the impact on students having a more robust sense of cultural competence and cultural safety, and, ultimately to reduced inequalities in health care and provision.

With regard to Shay's point (#3) about student voices, we agree. The problem, however, is that, if the curriculum doesn't address different worldviews, including those about the student–teacher relationship, then this silences voices, especially Indigenous ones.

Julia: The principle of respect among Pasifika communities impacts on Pasifika students seeking help and support. In my pastoral groups with Pasifika students, the psy disciplines exclude Pasifika worldviews (Rad et al., 2018) and, therefore, Pasifika students, who can feel a sense of not belonging in the course or programme. We think that, if courses and programmes and institutions were more transparent about their underlying philosophy, and Māori and Pasifika students were aware of this from the outset, then we could at least encourage authentic engagement including a respectful critique of psy models.

We also agree with Shay's point (#4) that any decolonised curriculum needs to challenge the dominant worldview; and, that this is not only a personal challenge and issue for some, even the majority of academics (as noted above), it is also a theoretical one. For instance, in its 50-year history, the *Journal of Curriculum Studies* has published four articles on racism and none on decolonisation. It is also a challenge for students.

Julia: Within a Pasifika worldview, our responsibilities are communal, which means that, alongside the student role, there are also family, church and community commitments. Often, these roles can be in direct conflict with each other, particularly when duties and obligations coincide with assessment deadlines and schedules. In addition to the demands of their studies, Māori and Pasifika students will have individual and collective duties across a number of domains such as culture (support to family in the islands), employment (to look after family), family (an older sibling caring for elders) and spiritual (church). Often when there is tension between these duties and roles, it is the individual role that is minimised, in this case, the student role. A decolonised or decolonisng curriculum and institution needs, therefore, to account for the practical implications of the worldviews by which students live.

With regard to power plays (Shay's point #5), we three agree that key to changing the curriculum (as well as the profession and the practitioner) is a redistribution of power, whether this involves power-sharing or, in some situations, people taking power (student protests, sit-ins, school refusals, etc.). Within an academic institution, this often involves having or getting a seat at the table, literally, being a member of a board of studies, an exam board or an academic board.

Keith: In my time in academia, I have been shocked at the amount of time spent by some colleagues resisting change. One particular Pākehā colleague almost boasted to me about how much he had done in advancing Māori psychology despite a distinct lack of evidence to the effect. When I and other colleagues proposed the development of some papers (courses) in psychology to address Māori and Pasifika worldviews, the same colleague lead the charge against this development (on the basis that I and my colleagues had not observed a specific piece of due process); five years later, no progress has been made.

Finally (on this), it is important to recognise that we cannot decolonise the curriculum without decolonising the academic institution and its systems (Shay's final point #6), including its expectations of staff.

Julia: As a Pasifika academic and psychologist, whilst we face similar challenges to our palagi friends and colleagues in academia to ensure we teach, research and publish, and contribute to leadership (or 'academic citizenship'), there is little acknowlegment in terms of our service to the community. For Pasifika, O le ala i le pule o le tautua, in order to lead one must serve. My service to the community is my acknowledgement of the principles of respect and reciprocity (Ioane, 2017). It is the community that has supported me to be where I am now, and it is the community that I shall continue to serve. Moreover, when we teach, we are constantly thinking about how our curriculum fits (or not) within Indigenous worldviews and how we introduce this respectfully. Similarly, whilst we have pressures to undertake research, we are careful to ensure that it can be applied to the communities that we serve; research has to have value to our community, otherwise it is purposeless. Our service to the community happens in many forms and at any time. It can mean membership on a board, mentoring of upcoming students, presentations at local community groups, participation in church or community events – often at short notice and with a high level of expectation from our communities. All this takes place alongside academic expectations and demands as well as our own cultural and family obligations, and none of this is genuinely acknowledged within academic expectations, standards or performance.

One important part of decolonising the institution and sharing power is – or would be – the appointment of more Māori and Pasifka academics. This is important not only for the staff concerned and the institution, but also for Māori and Pasifika students who need to recognise themselves in the lecturers by way of identity, worldviews, values and beliefs. This is made difficult if not impossible when Māori representation in the academic workforce is 5% (McAllister et al., 2019) (compared with 15.6% of the general population, as noted above), while Pasifika representation in the academic workforce is a mere 1.7% (Naepi, 2019) (compared with 7.4% of the general poulation and 15% of the population of Auckland: Statistics New Zealand, 2019).

Decolonising the profession

Whilst we might change the curriculum in the education and training for our psy disciplines, this does not mean that the profession as it is currently organised and operating will change. In this section, we briefly consider the issue of representation, which we view in the context of a commitment to Te Tiriti o Waitangi; and a 'mirror to society' argument and policy, which is concerned with equality (if not equity).

While the programme advisory boards and the boards or councils of the various psy professions may espouse their commitment to Māori, they tend to do so as another ethnic minority, and the specific relationship between Māori and Pasifika is usually ignored or minimised. Moreover, a review of the compostion of these boards and councils reveals a lack of key Māori and Pasifika representation (see New Zealand Psychologists Board, 2020; Psychotherapists Board of Aotearoa New Zealand, 2020), which reflects a more general problem of the very low numbers of Māori and Pasifika in senior leadership roles as seen in the health system (Came et al., 2020). One part of decolonising the psy professions would be for each and all of them to commit to honouring Te Tiriti o Waitangi.

Given the over-representation of Māori and Pasifika in adverse health and social statistics (as noted above), it is of concern that the people making the decisions are not representative of these vulnerable yet diverse communities. Significant and effective change can't happen if Māori and Pasifika aren't sitting at the table or are prevented from sitting at the table at which decisions are made, due to the failure of systems and policies, as well as the racism of colleagues. In order to change this, we suggest that, initially, a proportional 'mirror to society' policy (Crampton et al., 2012) is needed across the professions to ensure that equality, equity and diversity are not only held at a governance and strategic level, but are also a clear pathway to education/training, professional development and implementation. This will ensure that the selection of members to leadership and boards and councils will have, as part of our obligations to Te Tiriti o Waitangi, Māori representation, and, acknowledging the growing health disparities among Pasifika communities, also Pasifika representation: to influence improvements in health and well-being (Ministry of Health, 2020). It is important to note that the journey to address this particular inequity began in 1978 (Older, 1978) but, unfortunately, still continues (Scarf et al., 2019). Whatever the inadequacies of the curriculum by which practitioners were taught, as a profession, we must be open to and integrate the worldviews, practice, protocols and values of the communites that we serve.

Supporting the training, safety and development of Māori practitioners to work as Māori within the psy professions is essential. Levy (2018) has discussed the importance of building a critical mass of Māori psychologists in Aotearoa New Zealand, and there remains a high need for Māori psychologists across all sectors in which psychologists are employed and, specifically, to provide culturally meaningful and appropriate services to Māori. Current estimates of the Māori workforce put it at approximately 5% (Levy, 2018).

Indigenous or Māori psychology is also a growing area and a Kaupapa Māori scope of practice has been proposed by some as a method to recognise this area of expertise in practice (Levy, 2018). Indigenous psychology in Aotearoa New Zealand is based on Mātauranga Māori (Māori epistemologies) and prioritises and accepts Māori knowledge, values, beliefs and practices as valid and legitimate (Levy & Waitoki, 2015; Nikora, 2005). The goal of an Indigenous psychology is 'for Indigenous peoples to see their worldviews reflected back to them when they seek help for themselves, their families or their communities' (Waitoki et al., 2018, 178).

Finally, if these changes were to be implemented, how would we know if the new look psy professions were on track? Apart from increased numbers of Māori and Pasifika practitioners, relationships and partnerships are integral to Indigenous and ethnic minority communities (O'Carroll, 2013). In Aotearoa New Zealand, our experiences tell us that genuine partnerships with the community are effective to creating positive environments, so we suggest the formal establishment of relationships of the psy professions with iwi and church leaders as an example to measure the effectiveness of our services.

Decolonising the practitioner

Whatever one's experience of the curriculum of the professional education/training we studied, and whatever one's experience of the profession, practitioners have and retain the responsibility to practice safely, respectfully and effectively. In our experience, many practitioners in Aotearoa New Zealand lack disciplinary reflexivity, with the result that they continue to apply Western, individualistic notions of identifying problems, measuring outcomes and organising interventions, which for the most part do not fit Māori or other non-Pākeha cultures (Kirmayer, 2012). Indeed, in 2018, Dr Michelle Levy lodged a Treaty of Waitangi Tribunal claim *Wai2725 Psychology in Aotearoa* (Waitangi Tribunal, 2018) to highlight the Crown's failure to ensure psychology as an academic discipline, a profession and a practice meets the needs and demands of Māori. In this final section, we discuss three areas in which the Pākehā practitioner can be usefully decolonised: knowing about and engaging with Māori-led services; increasing their interaction with Māori communities; and being culturally safe and competent.

Supporting the training, safety and development of Māori practitioners to work as Māori within psy professions is essential. Levy (2018) has discussed the importance of building a critical mass of Māori psychologists in Aotearoa New Zealand. There remains a high need for Māori psychologists across all sectors in which psychologists are employed, particularly given the small but growing numbers of Māori in the profession; the current estimate of the Māori workforce is approximately 5%. A critical mass is needed to meet the needs of the population and to provide culturally meaningful and appropriate services to Māori. Indigenous or Māori psychology is also a growing area and a Kaupapa Māori scope of practice has been proposed by some as a method to recognise this area of expertise in practice (Levy, 2018). Indigenous psychology in Aotearoa is based on Mātauranga Māori (Māori epistemologies). It prioritises and accepts Māori knowledge, values, beliefs and practices as valid and legitimate (Levy & Waitoki, 2015; Nikora, 2005). The goal of an Indigenous psychology is 'for Indigenous peoples to see their worldviews reflected back to them when they seek help for themselves, their families or their communities' (Waitoki et al., 2018).

Many Māori-led services and Māori practitioners offer exemplars of how to work well with Māori. Whanaungatanga (building and maintaining connections and relationships) and manaakitanga (hospitality, uplifting mana or self-worth, status) are embedded in their practice and policies. The common threads of these practices is that they are holistic and centred on Māori understandings of wellness, are whānau centred, and emphasise the importance of spiritual as well as psychological and physical health; they also activate the potential of individuals and whānau, provide access to Māori culture and promote Māori aspirations to live well as Māori (Durie, 2011). Māori want the opportunity to experience their own strengths and success (Moewaka-Barnes et al., 2019). Advocacy and support for Māori and Māori practices by Pākehā and Tauiwi voices is vitally important to make the necessary changes in the system. Adequate resourcing of these initiatives is also vital to ensure that the benefits are sustained across multiple generations so that they can address inequities and enable ongoing transformation and self-determining futures in Aotearoa New Zealand. As part of a decolonising strategy for and of the practitioner, we place this first for two reasons: it honours what was here first; and it challenges the prioritising and privileging of settler-led 'mainstream' services.

A second step in decolonising practitioners and their practice is to prioritise the provision of services that are beneficial for Māori and so to increase interactions or encounters between Pākehā practitioners and Māori communities. Being in Māori environments provides the lived experience of practice such as whanaungatanga and manaakitanga in action. Such social interactions also provide an insight into the nuances of these behaviours, helping to deepen practitioners' understanding of Māori values and beliefs and how these are communicated and enacted (Pomare, 2015). Whanaungatanga is valued by Māori service users; the therapeutic relationship is known to have many benefits, and relational well-being is especially valued by Māori, Pasifika and many other collectivist cultures. Practitioners are often encouraged to introduce themselves with pepeha (a form of introduction that establishes identity and heritage, where significant geographical places are named), the purpose of which within Māori processes is to establish connections and to understand more about the person who is introducing themselves and where they come from. However, more emphasis is needed in practice on moving from simply reciting a pepeha to enacting whanaungatanga by looking for opportunities to make connections, utilising judicious self-disclosure and, thereby, reducing power differentials. This takes time, and, often, more time is needed to establish a genuine and authentic therapeutic alliance. Ongoing whanangatanga and engagement with the individual and whānau also enables positive outcomes.

Pikihuia: In my experience, amongst some Pākehā, there is a resistance to sharing and making connections due to concerns about maintaining privacy and keeping a distance between the professional and the service recipient. However, many Māori, Pasifika and other Indigenous practitioners are able to build and maintain culturally appropriate therapeutic relationships within ethical parameters and codes. There are also opportunities to extend manaakitanga by engaging in simple practices such as offering a service user a cup of tea, demonstrating care and also allowing of a gradual and natural flow into difficult conversations. Whilst time limitations are often cited as a reason for not being able to practice whanaungatanga and manaakitanga, the benefit of prioritising these is client and whānau satisfaction; increased engagement and reduced disengagement; cultural alignment; and an opportunity to utilise skills that are known to be therapeutic for Māori, Pasifika and other groups.

A third and important aspect of decolonising practitioners in Aotearoa New Zealand is to ensure that all practitioners are culturally safe and competent with regard to service recipients and whānau. Critical cultural awareness is often promoted as a first step for practitioners within the dominant Pākehā, Tau iwi culture, based on a view of the practitioner as a bearer of culture. As such, any intervention, regardless of how much it may be adapted by the practitioner, is a cultural artefact (Wendt & Gone, 2012). Humility and an openness to learning from Māori and other diverse cultures can provide a pathway to meaningful and effective work as well as reducing the possibility of harm. Black and Huygens (2016) offered some guidelines for working towards becoming a 'uniquely Pākehā psychologist in a culturally just relationship with Māori and other groups' (pp. 60–61) such as:

- Bearing in mind the European and American origins of psychological theories and practices, the cultural biases inherent in these and potential 'cultural danger' when applied to Māori and other cultures in research, therapy and community settings.
- Evaluating any assumptions that Western culture constitutes a superior culture.
- Affirming the epistemologies and methods of te ao Māori (the Māori world) and other cultural worlds.
- Consulting with and being accountable to senior cultural representatives, including having supervision.
- Opening up our disciplinary boundaries around cultural work. including recommendations made by Māori practitioners and experts.

Māori authors have also emphasised the importance of being informed by history, for example, learning about New Zealand history, colonisation and Te Tiriti o Waitangi – The Treaty of Waitangi (and knowing the differences between the two versions); and about the impact of historical trauma on Māori realities (Cooper, 2012). As long ago as 1993, Awatere-Huata challenged psychologists to learn about the Treaty and its impacts and to take action to making changes in practice and deconstructing systemic privilege. In this context, it is important that practitioners bring an equity lens to their mahi (work) that incorporates an analysis of power, taking into account social contexts of distress that are emphasised in the power threat meaning framework (Johnstone et al., 2018) and the Hauora/Meihana model (Pitama et al., 2017) which emphasises the importance of considering racism, marginalisation, colonisation and migration. Conceptualisations of behaviour that include an analysis of these factors can move us away from dehumanising clients and towards greater empathy for the people who receive our services.

***Pikihuia*:** In my experience as a person who has taught Māori perspectives to university students at both undergraduate and postgraduate levels and cultural competency training to registered professionals, there is still a lot of work to be done to begin to scratch the surface of getting practitioners to a level at which they can work effectively with Māori. Māori practitioners and teachers are often expected to push up against practitioners who have not been educated about New Zealand's colonial or Māori history, Te Tiriti o Waitangi, etc., and the requirement to become culturally competent practitioners is left to the motivation and good will of the individual. There is often no accountability to assess or measure whether a psychologist is fit to practice with Māori or other cultural groups outside of the dominant group. Māori practitioners and teachers often expend much of their energy educating non-Māori about privilege, discrimination and racism, and are frequently met with defensiveness and an unwillingness to acknowledge the realities or be open to change. The work of educating the dominant group about privilege and racism is tiring.

Kōrero whakamutunga – Conclusion

How do we make space for growth? Clearing away the old can enable us to see the strength of the pūtake (base/root) of the harakeke (flax bush) clearly. What does it mean to burn away the overgrowth? The clearing and burning off of old ways and attitudes is not easy. However, collective responsibility and committed action can ease the way forward.

Pikihuia: The work of Pākehā allies in this space is essential, for example, taking responsibility for educating the dominant group about privilege, prejudice, discrimination and racism so that Māori (and other marginalised groups) are able to direct our energies into Māori aspirations. As Durie (2011) wrote, Māori futures will be best served by Māori leadership and control.

With that in mind, we lay down a challenge. Let us support, provide for and give way to Māori leadership across education, health, justice, social, tamariki/mokopuna (child) protection and other related sectors. Let us truly acknowledge the partnership of Te Tiriti o Waitangi. Let us provide space for a 'mirror to society' policy where, for example, Pasifika communities genuinely influence both decision-making rocesses and practice and service outcomes. We call on the psy professions and practitioners to support Māori innovations; to disrupt social and economic harms to provide meaningful, effective and transformative services to Māori; and to help remove barriers (both internal and external) to enable success. Although we are critical of conservatism as well as reaction with our professions and colleagues, we are hopeful that there is a willingness and openness for change. If Western psychology and its psy professionals are willing to take an allied role, seeking service rather than colonial dominance, then it – and they – would be 'a good thing'. We draw on the wisdom and resilience of our tūpuna, their dreams and aspirations for us and plan for what we may also want for the future of our descendants.

E fofō le alämea, le alämea | Let the issues of the community be resolved by the community.

Kua takoto te mānuka | The mānuka leaves have been laid as a challenge to take up.

References

Anon. (1973). Therapy is change, not adjustment. *Radical Therapist, 3*(6). www.biblio.com/book/rough-times-formerlt-radical-therapist-volume/d/1362171780

Awatere-Huata, D. (1993). Challenges to psychology in Aotearoa. In L. W. Nikora (Ed.). *Cultural justice and ethics*. Waikato: National Standing Committee on Bicultural Issues, New Zealand Psychological Society.

Berry, J. W., Poortinga, Y. H., Segall, M. H., & Dasen, P. R. (2002). Psychology and the majority world. In J. W. Berry, Y. H. Poortinga, M. H. Segall, & P. R. Dasen

(Eds.). *Cross-cultural psychology: Research and applications.* (2nd ed., pp. 456–459). Cambridge: Cambridge University Press.

Black, R., & Huygens, I. (2016). Pākehā culture and psychology. In W Waitoki, J. S. Feather, N. R. Robertson, & J. J. Rucklidge (Eds.). *Professional practice of psychology in Aotearoa New Zealand* (3rd ed., pp. 49–66). Wellington: New Zealand Psychological Society.

Came, H., Badu, E., Ioane, J., Manson, L., & McCreanor, T. (2020). Ethnic (pay) disparities in public sector leadership from 2001–2016 in Aotearoa New Zealand. *International Journal of Critical Indigenous Studies, 13*(1), 70–85. https://doi.org/10.5204/ijcis.v13i1.1331

Connell, R. (2008). *Southern theory: The global dynamics of knowledge in social sciences.* Sydney: Allen & Unwin.

Cooper, E. (2012) Tōku reo, tōku ngākau: Learning the language of the heart. *Psychology Aotearoa, 64,* 97–103.

Crampton, P., Weaver, N., & Howard, A. (2012). Holding a mirror to society? The sociodemographic characteristics of the University of Otago's health professional students. *New Zealand Medical Journal, 125*(1361), 12–28. www.nzma.org.nz/journal/125–1361/5323/

Denny, A., Nielson, R, & Waititi, T. (2018, 5 April). Unknown Mortal Orchestra and Taika Waititi on New Zealand culture. *Dazed and Confused.* Retrieved from www.dazeddigital.com/music/article/39590/1/unknown-mortal-orchestra-ruban-nielson-taika-waititi-interview

Durie, M. (2011). *Nga tini whetu: Navigating Maori futures.* Wellington: Huia Publishers.

Elder, H., & Tapsell, R. (2013). Māori and the Mental Health Act. In J. Dawson & K. Gledhill (Eds.). *Mental Health Act in practice* (pp. 249–267). Victoria: Victoria University Press.

Fleming, P. (1984). The seven levels of listening and contribution training. In Pellin Centre, *Pellin Diploma course notes* (pp. 8–10). Available from the Pellin Centre, Avenue House, Tennyson Road, Kings Lynn, PE30 5PA, UK.

Howe, K. R. (Ed.) (2006). *Vaka Moana: Voyages of the ancestors. The discovery and settlement of the Pacific.* Auckland: David Bateman.

Ioane, J. (2017). Pasifika and psychology: Are we there yet. *Psychology Aotearoa, 9*(2), 70–77.

Ioane, J., & Lambie, I. (2016). Pacific youth and violent offending in Aotearoa New Zealand. *New Zealand Journal of Psychology, 45*(3), 23–29.

Levy, M. (2018). He Whiritaunoka: The Whanganui land report (Wai 2725). Retrieved from https://forms.justice.govt.nz/search/Documents/WT/wt_DOC_97551683/He%20Whiritaunoka%20Extracts.pdf

Levy, M., & Waitoki, W. (2015). Our voices, our futures: Indigenous psychology in Aotearoa New Zealand. In W. Waioki, J.S. Feather, N. R. Robertson & J. J Ruckliedge (Eds.). *Profesional practice of psychology in Aotearoa New Zealand* (3rd ed.; pp. 24–47). Wellington: New Zealand Psychological Society.

Johnstone, L. (2018). *The power threat meaning framework: Towards the identification of patterns in emotional distress, unusual experiences and troubled or troubling behaviour, as an alternative to functional psychiatric diagnosis.* London: British Psychological Society.

Kirmayer, L. J. (2012). Cultural competence and evidence-based practice in mental health: Epistemic communities and the politics of pluralism. *Social Science and Medicine, 75,* 249–256. doi: https://doi.org/10.1016/j.socscimed.2012.03.018

Marx, K. (1972). Theses on Feuerbach. In K. Marx, F. Engels, & V. Lenin *On historical materialism: A collection* (pp. 11–13). Moscow: Progress Publishers. (Original work published 1888.)

McAllister, T. G., Kidman, J., Rowley, O., & Theodore, R. F. (2019). *Why isn't my professor Māori? A snapshot of the academic workforce in New Zealand universities. MAI Review, 8*(2), 235–249.

Mikahere-Hall, A. (2020). Tūhono Māori: Promoting secure attachments for Indigenous Māori children. A conceptual paper. *Ata: Journal of Psychotherapy Aotearoa New Zealand, 23*(2), 49–59.

Ministry of Education. (2004). *Tertiary education strategy 2002–2007: Baseline monitoring report publication.* Wellington: Ministry of Education. www.educationcounts.govt.nz/publications/80898/tes/5659.

Ministry of Health. (2016). *Suicide facts: 2014 data.* Wellington: Ministry of Health.

Ministry of Health. (2020). *Ola Manuia: Pacific health and wellbeing action plan 2020–2025.* Wellington: Ministry of Health.

Moewaka Barnes, H., Henwood, W., Murray, J., Waiti, P., Pomare-Peita, M., Bercic, S., & McCreanor, T. (2019). Noho taiao: Reclaiming Māori science with young people. *Global Health Promotion, 26*, 35–43.

Naepi, S. (2019). Why isn't my professor Pasifika. A snapshot of the academic workforce in New Zealand universities. *MAI Journal*, 8, 219–234. doi: 10.20507/MAIJournal.2019.8.2.10

New Zealand Psychologists Board. (2020). Board members. Retrieved from www.psychologistsboard.org.nz/about-the-board2/board-members;

Nikora, L. W. (2005). *Māori and psychology: Indigenous psychology in New Zealand.* Waikato: Waikato University Māori and Psychology Research Unit.

O'Carroll, A. D. (2013). Virtual whanaungatanga: Māori utilizing social networking sites to attain and maintain relationships. *AlterNative: An International Journal of Indigenous Peoples, 9*(3), 230–245. https://doi.org/10.1177/117718011300900304

Office of the Children's Commissioner. (2020) *Pēpi Māori and the care and protection system.* Retrieved 31 August 2020, from www.occ.org.nz/publications/reports/pepi-maori-and-the-care-and-protection-system/

Older, J. (1978). *The Pākehā papers.* Dunedin: McIndoe.

Orange, D. (2012). Clinical hospitality: Welcoming the face of the devastated other. *Ata: Journal of Psychotherapy Aotearoa New Zealand, 16*(2), 165–178. https://doi.org/10.9791/ajpanz.2012.17

Pitama, S., Bennett, S., Waitoki, W., Valentine, H., Haitana, T., Pahina, J., & McLaughlan, A. (2017). Hauora Māori clinical guide for psychologists: Using the Hui process and the Meihana model in clinical assessment and formulation. *New Zealand Journal of Psychology, 46*(3), 7–13.

Pomare, P. (2015). He kākano ahau i ruia mai i rangiātea: Engaging Māori in culturally responsive child and adolescent mental health services. Doctorate of Clinical Psychology, University of Auckland, New Zealand.

Psychotherapy Board of Aotearoa New Zealand. (2020). Board members. Retrieved from www.pbanz.org.nz/index.php?BoardMembers

Rad, M. S., Martingano, A. J., & Ginges, J. (2018). Toward a psychology of Homo sapiens: Making psychological science more representative of the human population. *Proceedings of the National Academy of Sciences, 115*(45), 11401–11405. https://doi.org/10.1073/pnas.1721165115

The Radical Therapist Collective. (1971). Introduction. In *The radical therapist* (J. Agel, Producer; pp. ix–xxiii). New York: Ballantine Books.

Rogers, C. R. (1957). The necessary and sufficient conditions of therapeutic personality change. *Journal of Consulting Psychology, 21*, 95–103. https://doi.org/10.1037/h0045357

Rogers, C. R. (1959). A theory of therapy, personality and interpersonal relationships, as developed in the client-centered framework. In S. Koch (Ed.). *Psychology: A study of a science,* vol. 3, *Formulation of the person and the social context* (pp. 184–256). New York: McGraw-Hill.

Scarf, D., Waitoki, W., Chan, J., Britt, E., Nikora, L. W., Neha, T., & Hunter, J. A. (2019). Holding a mirror to society? Sociodemographic diversity within clinical psychology training programmes across Aotearoa. *New Zealand Medical Journal, 132*(1495), 79–81. Retrieved from https://assets-global.website-files.com/5e332a62c703f653182faf47/5e332a62c703f610e82fd439_Scarf-FINAL.pdf

Shay, S. (2016). Decolonising the curriculum: It's time for a strategy. *The Conversation*. Retrieved from https://worldpece.org/sites/default/files/artifacts/media/pdf/decolonising_the_curriculum-_its_time_for_a_strategy.pdf

Statistics New Zealand. (2019). 2018 census totals by topic. Retrieved from www.stats.govt.nz/information-releases/2018-census-totals-by-topic-national-highlights-updated

Theule, J., & Germain, S. (2017). Clinical psychology training in Canada and expectations for mobility: Is it time for change?. *Canadian Psychology/Psychologie canadienne, 58*(3), 288–291. https://doi.org/10.1037/cap0000112

Treaty2U. (2020). Te Tiriti o Waitangi | The Treaty of Waitangi. Retrieved from www.treaty2u.govt.nz/the-treaty-up-close/treaty-of-waitangi/

Tudor, K. (2012). Southern psychotherapies. *Psychotherapy and Politics International, 10*(2), 116–129. https://doi.org/10.1002/ppi.1265

Tudor, K. (2016). Raising (issues about) the banner: A critical reflection on New Zealand's flag debate (2015–2016). *Counterfutures: Left thought and practice Aotearoa, 2*, 83–112.

Tudor, K., & Begg, K. (2016). Radical therapy: A critical review. *Journal of Critical Psychology, Counselling and Psychotherapy*, 1–13.

Waitangi Tribunal. (2018). *WAI 2725 #1.1.1, The psychology in Aotearoa claim: Statement of claim.* https://waitangitribunal.govt.nz/treaty-of-waitangi/.

Waitoki, W., Dudgeon, P., & Nikora, L. W. (2018). Indigenous psychology in Aotearoa/New Zealand and Australia. In S. Fernando & R. Moodley (Eds.). *Global psychologies* (pp. 163–184). Basingstoke: Palgrave Macmillan.

Wendt, D. C., & Gone, J. P. (2012). Rethinking cultural competence: Insights from indigenous community treatment settings. *Transcultural Psychiatry, 49*, 206–222. DOI: https://doi.org/10.1177/1363461511425622

Wharewera-Mika, J. P., Cooper, E., Wiki, N., Field, T., Haitana, J., Toko, M., Edwards, E., & McKenna, B. (2016). Strategies to reduce the use of seclusion with tāngata whai I te ora (Māori mental health service users). *International Journal of Mental Health Nursing, 25*, 258–265. https://doi.org/10.1111/inm.12219

Woodard, W. (2014). Politics, psychotherapy, and the *1907 Tohunga Suppression Act. Psychotherapy and Politics International, 12*(1), 39–48. https://doi.org/10.1002/ppi.1321

Chapter 10

Counselling the 'other'

Cemil Egeli

Summary

This chapter explores the relevance of culture and the experience of being the 'other' in the world of counselling. It draws in theory and personal experience in its analysis of the counselling industry's approach to race.

Background and context

Counselling has a problem with race, ethnicity and culture.[1] Although there are no official figures, The Black African, Asian Therapy Network (BAATN, 2020) estimate that 5% of counsellors and psychotherapists in the UK are from Black and Ethnic Minority backgrounds, compared to BAME groups making up 12% of the population, indicating an inadequate level of representation.[2] Mertins-Brown (2018) observes that there is a lack of Black and BAME counsellors, whilst a disproportionate number of BAME people are forcibly admitted to and held within mental health hospitals. This is broadly supported by Bailey et al. (2018) who write that, within the counselling professions, it is widely regarded that there is a failure in training and education to address race. In a similar vein, Russell (2020) states that therapy training providers have a lack of understanding about race which means Black and minority ethnic trainees are more likely to experience trauma and drop out of courses.

The *Ethnic Inequalities in Mental Health Report* (Fitzpatrick et al., 2014) highlights key areas in which BAME people face barriers to mental health support. The findings are disturbing and include poor access to services and a recognition that BAME people are often at the end of harsh treatments and services. The report states that the biomedical model does not work and a psychosocial model is more effective. The Eurocentricity of therapeutic models plus the expert nature of the therapeutic relationship were cited as flaws in the biomedical model.

Although the British Association for Counselling and Psychotherapy (BACP) claims a commitment to equality (BACP, 2019) the organization appears to fetishize the biomedical model. This has been apparent in their current collaborative attempt to define and standardise counselling and psychotherapy, in which they reduced the ability to work culturally to a box-ticking exercise and elevated the status of the diagnostic medical model (Egeli, 2019). Their recent manifesto pledge (BACP, 2019a) appears to ideologically and linguistically align with the government's Improving Access to Psychological Therapies (IAPT) programme and colludes with the hegemony. IAPT, with its rigid and target-focused neoliberal framework does not have the flexibility to work with diverse communities (Boyles and McKinnon Fathi, 2019). It fosters a one size fits all approach which does not account for cultural differences. It also promotes individualism, manualised interventions and a managerialist culture (Loewenthal, 2018). The biomedical model puts an emphasis on evidence-based research, rooted in a positivist ontology which dehumanises people and reduces the complexity of human selves to statistics (Merrill and West, 2018). The medicalised model treats people as objects, involves social control of diverse groups and Western beliefs about mental health are seen to dominate other cultures globally (Watters, 2010; McNamara & Powell, 2020).

Despite the flaws of the neoliberal IAPT project, there is a view within the counselling professions that working within it could be a way of creating more therapeutic spaces for BAME people (Jackson, 2019). It seems that there is a failure to grasp that neoliberalism can be an oppressive form of neo-colonialism in itself. It enforces a stifling bureaucratic culture which isolates people within an interiorised understanding of self whilst promoting problematic binary categories of people (Thomas, 2019). These binaries are tied to colonial thinking which originally differentiated between colonisers and others (Lane, 2006).

According to Fernando (2012), the main difference between non-Western and Western approaches to mental health is the Western focus on individualism. This is rooted in colonial and enlightenment ideas and had racism at its core. Likewise Sue and Sue (2016) describe therapy as being individualistic and having an ethnocentric mono-culturalism which is dysfunctional and oppressive. They call for mental health workers to have a critical plurality to their work. The way ideas which underpin psychotherapeutic theories of personality have been (mis)used by colonialism cannot be ignored. The self-actualising tendency was originally reserved for what was seen as superior enlightened Western humans as opposed to inferior others, whilst Freudian theories were used to create a sense of othering non-Western peoples (Tuhiwai Smith, 2012) and influenced colonial anthropological thought, helping to create the trope of the primitive savage (Torgovnik, 1990). As Fernando (2012) suggests, we are left with a legacy of 'race thinking' (and the accompanying racism), which still impacts psychological therapies today.

Moodley and West (2005) state that, as they stand, counselling and psychotherapy are too individualistic and Eurocentric, rendering minorities as outsiders. Furedi (2004) argues that the individualistic nature of therapy distances us from each other, this is in opposition to non-Western concepts such as 'I am because we are' (More, 2004, 157) reflecting a more collectivist philosophy of solidarity. There can be a place of balance between the individual and the collective, as to separate the two entirely could be another binary division. Francis (2018) suggests, the two can work together, as individual voices can be expressed within a collective logic. The concept of self-actualisation, for instance, can be both individual and social (Tuhiwai Smith, 2012). Tudor (2018, 52) makes the case that Western thinkers articulate what he calls '"We" psychology', arguing that psychotherapeutic theories are compatible with collectivist ideas. As Nolan and West (2019) suggest, we can have interconnectedness in our individual meaning making. In my research into cultural experiences there is a place for the individual; relational and social. Identity is continuously negotiated in our personal interactions with others and the wider society (Orbe and Harris, 2015). Individual stories are 'redolent with the collective' (Merrill & West, 2009, 68). However, to therapeutically enforce an individualistic perspective on a client would be to deny their social context, culture and experience.

A growing culturally mixed new wave – the new 'other'

People who are of a mixed background are one of the fastest growing populations in the UK (ONS, 2019). Jivraj (2012) states that mixed ethnic identity had grown by 80% in the 2000s and that included over 1 million people. These trends are apparent in the USA where the US Census Bureau in 2012 reported that the multiple-race population grew faster than the single race population. However, it is difficult to capture the subtleties and nuances of cultural identity within census categories (Egeli, 2017). I often wonder which box to tick in ethnicity questionnaires and opt for the 'other' category and I am mindful that extreme forms of 'other other' were used during apartheid in South Africa (Moodley, 2003). I sometimes feel othered within BAME discourse as I do not fit a specific ethnic category. Counselling as a profession seems to be stuck working within very fixed racialised paradigms, rooted in binary and dichotomised thinking (Moodley, 2003; Altman, 2006); there is a growing culturally mixed new wave which is being ignored in the discourse. The new 'other'. The mixed 'other'.

My story – autoethnography

I am of mixed culture. My father is Turkish and my mother is English. I am fair-skinned in appearance and often perceived as monoculturally white-English, as such I experience some invisibility as an ethnic minority.

This originally motivated me to undertake a study of myself in the form of autoethnography which was based on my mixed cultural heritage (Egeli, 2015; Egeli, 2016; Egeli, 2017). I wanted to capture the complexity and fluidity of my experience which was not fully reflected in the academic literature or in professional practice discourse (Moodley, 2007).

The method itself challenges binary divides, dominant discourses and the bio-medical perspective (Allen-Collinson, 2013). I resonated with Bochner (1997,

424) who wanted to invite engagement with the 'particularities of the experience' rather than be stuck with theories, categories or labels. Autoethnography allowed me to challenge the labels I have found so oppressive and unhelpful whilst connecting the personal to the social and political (Ellis, 2004).

I adopted a creative approach to writing my study, weaving narrative and vignettes (including extracts based on journals in italics) together with some analysis (Humphries, 2005; Egeli, 2017). I present and revisit some extracts here which come under themes: language, appearance, name, circumcision and Brexit.

Language

I spent my early childhood growing up in Turkey, the only person I spoke English to was my mum. She had been afraid that I was going to lose my English language and I wonder if I absorbed some of those fears. Turkish was my first language but English was my mother's language.

On returning to Britain I did not continue to speak Turkish and lost my language. This gave me a sense of loss but also personal failure which was easy to forget when in England. No one spoke Turkish, it was not seen as relevant. People would say that I was better off learning French as it was more useful. That hurt. I am not French.

I spent many summers in Turkey listening to family and friends, understanding conversations but not being fully able to join in. People would look to others for a response. I could not speak for myself, I was embarrassed. I knew what they were saying but I couldn't clearly articulate myself. I had moved from being a fluent bilingual child, to being silenced and verbally debilitated. Burman (2008) recognises the emotional significance of language tied in with cultural and national identification. In my case I had been swept away from my Turkish home and family whom I loved. My dad for that period had to remain in Turkey due to military commitments. I had been thrown into a new world, had to negotiate linguistic change and had suffered a loss of my Turkish life. Language was a big part of my loss, trauma and grief (Priven, 2008).

Over the years I have struggled with loss and the centrality of language:

> A Turkish friend of mine died unexpectedly. I found out on social media through the bits of Turkish I could understand on their profile page. I wasn't sure at first, it seemed too horrific to be true, but I soon began to realise, mainly due to the photos that had been posted. I wanted to know what happened and tell people I was sorry and sad. I got direct messages, written in Turkish from their friends and family, perhaps seeing my name they thought I could correspond, but I couldn't reach out in the moment – I was left alienated and alone in grief. I sent my condolences in English but it's not what I really wanted to say. (2017)
>
> I was visiting London, a Turkish lady had a small child who was running around. I could understand every word she said to her child, things my

> family had said to me. The child came running over to me talking and I could not respond. She shouted at her child to leave me alone, I smiled and nodded. I wanted to say something smart or funny, a casual colloquial comment but couldn't. I wanted her to know that I knew, but I couldn't say anything. My biggest fear was being wrong, being an imposter, a failed Turk.
>
> (2015)

The way a person uses language is an observable aspect of their cultural identity (McLeod, 2009), language proficiency playing a role in identity development (Phinney et al., 2001). Aydingün & Aydingün (2004) suggest that the links between Turkish identity and language are particularly strong and are symbolic of the culture. My own identity was tied in with my language and was gagged by my new dominant culture. I have felt attracted to and torn between two languages which have held different meanings for me, I have also faced self-doubt not feeling I can speak either of my native languages well enough (Firmat, 2005).

Freely (2014) observes that the Turkish language has emotional undercurrents which the words conceal. Whenever I hear Turkish, it sounds musical; I get it. I hear the inflections. I understand something beyond the words and it is that something I cannot always respond to verbally.

> A local bar in Izmir had a resident band that played Turkish music. I knew I could play along so I asked to play and joined in on violin … here I was on stage with a Turkish crowd and my family were there too. I got a burst of adrenaline and language did not matter, something opened up and was flowing through my fingers, here I was connecting with a largely Turkish audience and in that moment saying everything I had ever wanted to through music … Turkish music.
>
> (2015)

Appearance

> You don't look Turkish. You are not what I expected.

Two phrases I am continually experiencing throughout my life. Some people make assumptions of me based on my skin colour, my name as they hear it on the phone and as they see it written down. I always explain that I am half Turkish and half English. A lifetime of being half and not whole.

> After surgery a nurse said to me, 'Now I am going to say to you something people have said to me all my life … You don't look Turkish.' He had an Italian dad and an Italian name. He told me that throughout his life people had told him he did not look Italian. He had red hair. His comment is so healing. There is someone out there like me.
>
> (2015)

It feels as if my heritage is constantly examined and questioned,

> I feel people look closely at me for signs of difference. Many have said, 'Oh yes, I can see you have a Turkish nose!' What does a Turkish nose look like?
>
> (2018)

In Turkey people do not accept my heritage; I have been called 'white cheese' and some Turks have refused to accept that I was in any way Turkish even though I had lived there years before they were born. People seem to form physical expectations of me based on my name.

> I remember working with a journalist from a national newspaper. We had spent much time on the phone. She came into the office and declared: 'I thought you were an Arab boy!' similarly when I met a famous comedian, he declared, 'I thought you were an Asian lad, I left my Asian jokes at home!'
>
> (2014)
>
> 'You are not what I imagined' said someone interviewing me at a work agency. I am angry! What does he imagine? Who did he expect?
>
> (2014)

There even seem to be expectations of my children:

> Returning from the Netherlands my family were stopped at UK customs. The official asked 'Why do your children have blonde hair? You have Turkish names', we had to prove we were their parents. I was taken aback, it felt like a hostile environment.
>
> (2019)

Being fair-skinned has rendered a part of me as being invisible and as a result I have struggled to feel valid as a person of two cultures. The assumption has been made on both sides that I don't 'look' Turkish. This may have triggered initial internal conflicts about my external appearance (Katz, 1996). I face perceptions from other people on a daily basis and whilst I feel angry about it I wonder if I am angry because I may believe these stereotypes myself. As I do not appear what people may think is obviously foreign, that seems to give licence to people to say anything they choose. As I may appear English, they perhaps feel they cannot offend. I am repeatedly reminded of my ambiguity. Would people say I don't look English?

> I was attending counselling training on anti-discriminatory practice. Someone suggested I may not be ethnic enough to work with ethnic clients. I felt discriminated against by some forms of anti-discriminatory practise and rhetoric. I did not feel included within it.
>
> (2015)

Yomtoob (2014) talks of living within multiple identity locations and is hurt by misrecognitions which occur through stereotyping. Similarly Fouad (2001) describes one of her central struggles as negotiating the conflicting expectations of other people's attributions of cultures. Like Fouad, I am often perceived to be from a dominant white and majority culture but echoing Hector (in Ellis, 2004, 240–244), who is Latino and White, I feel delegitimized as an ethnic minority and have no other voice other than an English person. Inside there is a Turkish person that is not validated (and suppressed by others). I have not consciously ever felt as fully English as many people from both countries repeatedly tell me I am.

> … our visit to Turkey was coming to an end so me and my brother went to a local cafe to get some fresh lokma (doughnuts). The owner refused to serve us, they had not wanted to serve who they thought were two English youths. My dad was angry, he shouted at the owner, 'THEY ARE TURKS!' … this was all the validation I needed.
>
> (2015)

Name

> I have had difficulty saying my name. I cannot say it in England with a Turkish accent so it gets morphed or Anglicised into sounding phonetically different to the extent that Turkish people sometimes don't understand my name.
>
> (2014)

I often have to explain my name when meeting someone new. It is spelt with a C but pronounced as a J. It felt isolating as a child as I never saw my name written down anywhere. I remember reading Eric Kastner's children's book *Emil and the Detectives* and going through the whole book putting a C before the name Emil to make CEmil. This was about belonging (May, 2013).

People have perceptions of me based on my name. When they meet me I may not live up to expectations. On paper they often see the C and believe my name to be either Welsh or Polish; on the phone they think I am Asian or Arab. In some instances my name is also seen as being female.

> I remember shortly after 9/11 I was corresponding with people in New York. As the dust settled from the awful attacks, there seemed to be a new hostility. I became acutely aware of having a Muslim name. Someone asked where it was from and I joked, it's one of those silly European names. I was feeling a tension I had not felt before.
>
> (2015)

Khosravi (2012) remarks that names have strong ethnic and religious connotations and within Sweden there has been anti-Muslim sentiment. These are sentiments I have felt in regards to my name. Whilst working for a counselling organisation, I heard some potential clients refused to see me because of my name. A counsellor told me that clients were free to choose who they want but this felt like discrimination.

> People are judging me … they don't know me but are making a judgement based on a name. When I go to A&E in agony, I don't give a shit who treats me, I just need help with my pain … how much help do these people really want? Fuck counsellor/client ethnic matching, who knows who anybody is? (2014)
>
> I thought you might be a white Jihadi … someone said.
>
> (2019)

My name has given me some visibility. It has been important in constructing a cultural sense of who I am (Dion, 1983). Kim & Lee (2011) state that naming provides important information about ethnicity, kinship and gender. In my case it has not helped provide that information to people all of the time. The perceptions people have had of my name have conflicted with the perceptions of my physicality (Pilcher, 2016). On the phone some people do not believe I am English, in person they do not believe I am a Turk, fuelling my identity conflicts.

> I was doing temporary office work at a gas company, I often encountered prejudice on the phone, people questioned my English and the ability to fill in forms, my team leader took me to one side and said, 'Can't you get a proper name?, Why don't you call yourself Jimmy or something?' I left shortly after that. I felt I couldn't complain as I was just too English.
>
> (2015)

Rites of passage

In Turkey circumcision (known as sünnet) is an important rite of passage for Turkish boys, symbolically marking their entry into manhood (Rizarlar et al., 2017). Unlike in the West it is not performed during the neonatal period but later in childhood (Şahin et al., 2003). Growing up I would regularly see other little boys ritually dressed as mini Ottoman sultans or princes with crowns, fur-lined capes and white silky suits ready for their ceremonies. Some would go past in open top cars with the live music of screaming zurnas and banging drums. It was exciting but terrifying too.

> I remember one time seeing two boys in their princely outfits arriving at a building and being taken for their circumcision. It didn't take long before they came out. I will never forget the tears and the agony on the face of one of them, they could barely walk, they stumbled off in silence. I was wondered when my time would come.
>
> (2018)

I would hear of friends and family members having the cut. It was always described as a cut. I wasn't sure what that meant but I knew that to be a man you needed to be cut. I sensed some family tensions around it.

> As a teenager I was at a party in Turkey, and a lady asked if I had been done. I shook my head, saying 'not yet'. The party fell silent, everyone looked and laughed.
>
> (2018)

In the film *East is East* (1999) it is revealed that the youngest member of a mixed cultural family (Sajid) had not been circumcised. His mum's friend inspects him to reveal 'It's still there!' (his foreskin). His discomfort is clear in the film and it chimed with me as it related specifically to a mixed cultural experience.

A psychodynamic interpretation may reveal a castration anxiety associated with the fear and trauma of circumcision, the actual act itself helping to resolve the issue perhaps forming part of a cultural road map to masculinity (Canserver, 1965; Crapanzano, 1980; Sahin, 2003). More socially, Punzi (2014), relating to Jews, writes that if you do not cut off your foreskin you are cut off from your people and it is inherently connected to male identity. Öztürk (1973) highlights the fact that circumcision works within a societal framework to integrate one's self-concept, body image and sexuality. He talks of Turkish people associating with feelings of shame and defectiveness if they have not had the procedure. My experiences reflect some of these ideas. I felt the fear but didn't transform it through the ritual and it had an impact on my own sense of self and masculinity. Rituals may foster a sense of belonging and help us to order our biographies in the symbolic world we live in (Berger & Luckman, 1966) and mark a transitory or liminal passage from one age to another (Van Gennep, 1960). However, coming from two cultures made it difficult, I was in a constant state of liminal flux. I was operating between social structures, my liminality being a state in itself rather than a stage within a rite of passage (Hall, 1991). The ritual may have helped resolve a sense of belonging or identity within one culture but perhaps not the other.

Whilst I missed out on Islamic and cultural rites in Turkey, in England I took Christian rites of baptism and confirmation. I felt torn between religions.

> I was somewhat reassured by the idea that St Paul and the New Testament said I didn't have to be circumcised although I was envious of the fact that Jesus had been – he was ok, at least he had fulfilled his covenant with God.
>
> (2018)

Brexit

Brexit has helped to create divisive and oversimplified categories of race and migration that have invoked colonial prejudices and sparked a rise in hate crimes (Burrell et al., 2019). During the UK Brexit campaign, I remember driving along and seeing a 'vote leave' poster which said:

> TURKEY
> (population 76 million)
> **IS JOINING THE EU**
> **Vote leave, take back control**

I was shocked and had to pull over. I shouted out loud to myself, 'WE ARE ALREADY HERE!' As a Turk I felt excluded by what appeared to be the elitist Christian capitalist club that is the European Union (EU). Now I was being used as a fear-mongering trope for the 'vote leave' campaign. I knew Turkey were not joining any time soon and this was racist propaganda. It was playing on tropes of the Turks threatening Europe, the idea of the 'Ottoman peril' (Said, 2003) still used in EU political discourse today (Karlsson, 2006; Nugent, 2007). Whilst there are debates about Turkish identity (Dudley, 2015), Turkey is seen as different from the European mainstream, culture and religion being a part of that (Nugent, 2007). For years I have witnessed what Carter (1995) describes as the inferiority paradigm which is grounded in Western colonialism and is the belief that groups other than Europeans were inferior. I have also experienced an attitude of a British civilised 'norm' which marginalises other groups and is rooted in a sense of orientalism (Modood, 1997; Said, 2003). I have heard Turks described by terms such as barbaric, backward, brutal, animals, dirty, thugs, savages, unevolved, greasy, slimey. Often to my face and sometimes said in a very British and innocuous way.

All the otherness I had felt was now encapsulated in a poster which demonstrated a malicious form of anti-Turkism. It played into fixed and simplistic definitions of what cultural identity is, as the media and press persistently do. It tapped into the internal tensions and oppressions I have felt for years. It stung. This was political.

Implications for counselling

This chapter explores some of my process as I experienced at different times, which is a complex interplay of different intersecting factors. I hope it can help readers to remain open to the varying possibilities of cultural experience and help them to see beyond some of the limiting discourses and stereotypes that define people's identity and lived experiences (Diamond & Gillis, 2006). It is important to recognise the new mixed other, the growing mixed demographic as our society and world moves beyond binaries and fixed simplistic definitions of race, ethnicity and culture. The counselling world radically needs to catch up with cultural developments.

Education/training

It was counselling training which brought to my self-awareness some of the wider challenges and inner tensions I have faced as a person of mixed cultural heritage. This was partly down to the transformative and experiential nature of the pedagogy which helped to shift my consciousness and understanding of my sense of self (Drirkx, 2012). Working culturally cannot be reduced to a tick box on a competency framework, to do that would be to collude with colonial and binary thinking. Educating for critical consciousness could be a good starting point (Freire, 1974/2013). It may help us to understand our own positionality within various social and cultural structures with which we can explore our differences and essential sameness (Dudgeon et al., 2018).

Therapeutic practice

Moodley (2007) called for multicultural counselling to be reframed within a fluid third space where a multiplicity of cultures can converge, calling for the inclusion of white people as multicultural clients. Fouad (2001) wrote that we need to acknowledge there are many people who are products of multiple worlds and cultures; cultural diversity is not just about visible ethnicity. The way I appear, be it in person, on the phone, online or on paper, is not necessarily a reflection of my experience. Our clients can experience this too. I would urge us to challenge the cultural assumptions we may make about people. As a culturally mixed person I do not fit the boxes ascribed to me. I do wonder if there could be a more covert racism within the counselling profession which does not necessarily apply to visible difference?

This leads me to ask questions of potential ethnic matching with clients and counsellors. I wonder where I may fit in this discourse. Would I be considered English, Turkish or ethnic enough to work with clients? Would judgments be made on my appearance? As a counsellor I also wonder how much I need to disclose about my cultural background to clients who may be forming assumptions based on my name.

In light of the current changing society we live in, Nolan and West (2019) have called to extend horizons within therapy to include perspectives from the liminal edges of experience, whilst Macdonald (2019) challenges fixed definitions of culture, exploring the idea of a metaculture which is universal to all, amidst the myriad of competing discourses. Perhaps we need to encourage integrative ways of working which can accommodate a plurality of perspectives and work alongside or even challenge conventional counselling paradigms. This could include spiritual or indigenous practices (Moodley and West, 2005). The danger for the counselling world is the neoliberal march towards manualised and standardised biomedical paradigms, which are not helpful for working culturally. They reinforce attitudes which are oppressive.

If we are to support the growing demographic of culturally mixed people as therapists we need a nuanced awareness and enhanced understanding of these experiences. More qualitative research and sharing biographical and autoethnographic stories can help us explore the commonalities of human experience which can challenge binary, hegemonic and colonial thinking whilst giving a space for marginal voices. The voices of the culturally mixed new wave, the new other.

Notes

1 The terms race, ethnicity and culture have differing social and political implications. They are used interchangeably in counselling and psychotherapy literature whilst still essentially exploring the same issues relating to cultural identity in the counselling process (McLeod, 2009). I refer to the terms race and ethnicity as social constructs rather than fixed realities (Tuckwell, 2002) and personally prefer to use the term culture as it covers a wide spectrum of experience, my ethnicity perhaps being a part of it.

2 It is important to note that the acronym BAME is problematic as it can, in itself, be labelling and othering (Cousins, 2019). I refer to it in this chapter in relation to current discourses that use it.

References

Ali, S. (2003). *Mixed-race: Post-race*. Oxford: Berg.

Allen-Collinson, J. (2013). Autoethnography as the engagement of self/other, self/culture, self/politics, and selves/futures. In S. Holman-Jones, T. Adams & C. Ellis (Eds.). *Handbook of autoethnography* (pp. 281–299). London: Routledge.

Altman, N. (2006). Black and white thinking: A psychoanalyst reconsiders race. In R. Moodley & S. Palmer (Eds.). *Race, culture and psychotherapy – Critical perspectives in multicultural practice* (pp. 139–149). London: Routledge.

Aydingün, A., & Aydingün, I. (2004). The role of language in the formation of Turkish national identity and Turkishness. *Nationalism and Ethnic Politics, 10*(3), 415–432 doi:10.1080/13537110490518264

BAATN (2020). Personal communication.

BACP (2019a). GE 2019 – Manifesto submission [online]. Available from: www.bacp.co.uk/media/7063/bacp-ge2019-manifesto-submission.pdf

BACP (2019b). Our commitment to equality [online]. Available from: www.bacp.co.uk/careers/work-for-bacp/equality-and-diversity/

Bailey, N., George, H., Khan, M., Jackson, C., & Weaver, D. (2018). Editor's note. *Therapy Today, 29*(8), 3.

Berger, P., & Luckman, T. (1966). *The social construction of reality: A treatise in the sociology of knowledge.* London: Penguin.

Bochner, A. P. (1997). It's about time: Narrative and the divided self. *Qualitative Inquiry, 3*(4), 418–438.

Boyles, J., and McKinnon, F. (2019). At what cost? The impact of IAPT on third-sector psychological therapy provision. In C. Jackson & R. Rizq (Eds.). *The industrialisation of care: Counselling, psychotherapy and the impact of IAPT* (pp. 232–252). Monmouth: PCCS Books.

Burman, E. (2008). *Deconstructing developmental psychology*. 2nd ed. London: Routledge.

Burrell, K., Hopkins, P., Isakjee, A., Lorne, C., Nagel, C., Finlay, R., & Rogaly, B. (2019). Brexit, race and migration. *Environment and Planning C: Politics and Space, 37*(1), 3–40. doi:10.1177/0263774X18811923

Cansever, G. (1965). Psychological effects of circumcision. *British Journal of Medical Psychology, 38*, 321–331. doi: /10.1111/j.2044-8341.1965.tb01314.x

Carter, R. T. (1995). *The influence of race and racial identity in psychotherapy: Toward a racially inclusive model.* New York: John Wiley & Sons.

Cousins, S. (2019). *Overcoming every day racism: Building resilience and wellbeing in the face of discrimination and micro-aggressions.* London: Jessica Kingsley Publishers.

Crapanzano, V. (1980). Rite of return: Circumcision in Morocco. In W. Muensterberger & L. Bryce Boyer (Eds.). *The psychoanalytic study of society* (vol. 9, pp. 15–36). New York: Psychohistory Press.

Diamond, S. L., & Gillis, J. R. (2006). Approaching multiple diversity: Addressing the intersections of class, gender, sexual orientation and different abilities. In C. Lago (Ed.). *Race, culture and counselling: The ongoing challenge,* 2nd ed. (pp. 217–228). Maidenhead: Open University Press.

Dion, K. (1983). Names, identity and self. *Names: A Journal of Onomastics, 31*(4), 245–257. doi:10.1179/nam.1983.31.4.245

Dirkx, J. M. (2012). Self-formation and transformative learning: A response to 'Calling transformative learning into question: Some mutinous thoughts', by Michael Newman. *Adult Education Quarterly,* 62(4), 399–405. doi:10.1177/0741713612456420

Dudgeon, P. Darlaston-Jones, D. & Bray, A. (2018). Teaching indigenous psychology: A conscientisation, de-colonisation and psychological literacy approach to curriculum. In C. Newnes & L. Golding (Eds.). *Teaching critical psychology: International perspectives* (pp. 123–147). London: Routledge.

Dudley, D. (2015). Identity crisis: Turkey, Europe, and Erdoğan. Available at: www.businessweekme.com/Bloomberg/newsmid/190/newsid/599

East is East (1999). Directed by Damien O'Donnell. Written by Ayub Khan-Din, 'Sajid has a foreskin'. Available at: www.youtube.com/watch?v=2UDtinc9lLU

Egeli, C. (2015). An individual experience of the impact of a mixed cultural heritage, an autoethnographic study. MA Dissertation. University of Manchester.

Egeli, C. (2016). I'm half Turkish – dancing bears and marble stairs. *Journal of Critical Psychology Counselling and Psychotherapy, 16*(4), 245–256. http://hdl.handle.net/10034/620568 1471-7646

Egeli, C. (2017). Autoethnography: A methodological chat with self. *Counselling Psychology Review, 32*(1), 5–15.

Egeli, C. (2019). Counselling and psychotherapy: Hierarchies, epistemicide and bad medicine. *Clinical Psychology Forum, 318*, 17–20.

Ellis, C. (2004). *The ethnographic I: A methodological novel about autoethnography.* Lanham, MD: AltaMira Press.

Fernando, S. (2012). Race and culture issues in mental health and some thoughts on ethnic identity. *Counselling Psychology Quarterly, 25*(2), 113–123. doi:10.1080/09515070.2012.674299

Firmat, G. P. (2005). On bilingualism and its discontents. *Daedalus,* Summer, *134*(3), 89–92. doi: 10.1162/0011526054622114

Fitzpatrick, R., Kumar, S., Ohemaa Nkansa-Dwamena, O., and Thorne, L. (2014). *Ethnic inequalities in mental health: Promoting lasting positive change. Report of findings.*

London: LankellyChase Foundation, Mind, The Afiya Trust and Centre for Mental Health. https://lankellychase.org.uk/wp-content/uploads/2015/07/Ethnic-Inequality-in-Mental-Health-Confluence-Full-Report-March2014.pdf.

Fouad, N. A. (2001). Reflections of a nonvisible racial/ethnic minority. In J. G. Ponterotto, J. M. Casas, L. A. Suzuki & C.M. Alexander (Eds.). *Handbook of multicultural counselling,* 2nd ed. (pp. 55–63). London: Sage.

Francis, S. (2018). The political economy of the southern Kalahari. Paper presented at the Social Science research seminar, University of Chester, April.

Freely, M. (2014). *Angry in Piraeus.* Paris: Sylph Editions, Centre for Writers & Translators, American University of Paris.

Freire, P. (1974/2013). *Education for critical consciousness.* London: Bloomsbury.

Furedi, F. (2004). *Therapy culture: Cultivating vulnerability in an uncertain age.* London: Routledge.

Gonzales-Backen, M. A., & Unmans' a-Taylor, A. J. (2011). Examining the role of physical appearance in Latino adolescents' ethnic identity. *Journal of Adolescence, 34,* 151–162. doi.org/10.1016/j.adolescence.2010.01.002

Hall, J. (1991). The watcher at the gates of dawn: The transformation of self in liminality and by the transcendent function. In N. Scwartz-Salant & M. Stein (Eds.). *Liminality and transitional phenomena* (pp. 33–51). Asheville, NC: Chiron Publications.

Humphries, M. (2005). Getting personal: Reflexivity and autoethnographic vignettes. *Qualitative Inquiry, 11,* 840. doi:10.1177/1077800404269425

Jackson, C. (2019). Black spaces, Black faces. *Therapy Today, 30*(8), 20–24.

Jivraj, S. (2012). Dynamics of diversity (evidence from the 2011 census). Manchester University prepared by ESRC as part of CoDE.

Karlsson, I. (2006). The Turk as a threat and Europe's 'Other'. *International Issues and Slovak Foreign Policy Affairs, 15*(1), 62–72. www.jstor.org/stable/26590546

Katz, I. (1996). *The construction of racial identity in children of mixed parentage: Mixed metaphors.* London: Jessica Kingsley Publishers.

Khosravi, S. (2012). White masks/Muslim names: Immigrants and name-changing in Sweden. *Race and Class, 53*(3): 65–80. doi.org/10.1177/0306396811425986

Kim, J., & Lee, K. (2011). 'What's your name?' Names, naming practices, and contextualized selves of young Korean American children. *Journal of Research in Childhood Education, 25*(3), 211–227. doi: 10.1080/02568543.2011.579854

Kinross, L. (1964). *Atatürk: The rebirth of a nation.* London: Weidenfeld & Nicolson.

Lane, R. (2006). *The postcolonial novel.* Cambridge: Polity Press.

Loewenthal, D. (2018). IAPT: Also promoting individualism at the expense of the common good? *European Journal of Psychotherapy and Counselling, 20*(3), 249–256. doi: 10.1080/13642537.2018.1495300

MacDonald, G. (2019). Culture as a resource in the creation of meaning: Part one. In G. Nolan and W. West (Eds.). *Extending horizons in helping and caring therapies: Beyond the liminal in the healing encounter* (pp. 92–105). London: Routledge.

May, V. (2013). *Connecting self to society: Belonging in a changing world.* Basingstoke: Palgrave Macmillan.

McLeod, J. (2009). *An Introduction to Counselling* (4th ed.). Maidenhead: McGraw Hill.

McNamara, B. and Powell, J. (2020). The rise of psychiatry: Mental illness/disorder and social control. In P. Taylor, S. Morely & J. Powell (Eds.). *Mental health and punishment* (pp. 6–19). London: Routledge.

Mertins-Brown, W. (2018). Come on, people, hear me! *Therapy Today, 29*(8), 26–27.

Merrill, B., & West, L. (2009). *Using biographical methods in social research*. London: SAGE.

Merrill, B., & West, L. (2018). A history of biographical research in the United Kingdom. *Revista Brasileira de pesquisa (auto)biográfica, 3*(9), 765–780. https://www.revistas.uneb.br/index.php/rbpab/article/view/5588

Modood, T., & Werner, N. (Eds.). (1997) *Debating cultural hybridity: Multi-cultural identities and the politics of anti-racism*. London: Zed Books.

Moodley, R. (2003). Matrices in black and white: Implications of cultural multiplicity for research in counselling and psychotherapy. *Counselling and Psychotherapy Research: Linking Research with Practice, 3*(2), 115–121. doi.org/10.1080/14733140312331384482

Moodley, R. (2007). (Re)placing multiculturalism in counselling and psychotherapy. *British Journal of Guidance and Counselling, 35*(1), 1–22. doi.org/10.1080/03069880601106740

Moodley, R., and West, W. (Eds.) (2005). *Integrating traditional healing practices into counselling and psychotherapy.* London: Sage.

More, M. P. (2004). Philosophy in South Africa under and after apartheid. In W. E. Abraham, A. Irele & I. A. Menkiti (Eds.). *A companion to African philosophy* (pp. 149–161). Oxford: Blackwell.

Nolan, G., & West, W. (2019). *Extending horizons in helping and caring therapies: Beyond the liminal in the healing encounter.* London: Routledge.

Nugent, N. (2007). The EU's response to Turkey's membership application: Not just a weighing of costs and benefits. *Journal of European Integration, 29*(4), 481–502. https://doi.org/10.1080/07036330701502480

ONS (2019). Nomis official labour market statistics. Available from: www.nomisweb.co.uk/census/2011.

Orbe, M. P., & Harris, T. M. (2015). *Interracial communication: Theory into practice,* 3rd ed. Los Angeles, CA: Sage.

Öztürk, O. M. (1973). Ritual circumcision and castration anxiety. *Psychiatry, 36*(1), 49. doi/abs/10.1080/00332747.1973.11023745

Phinney, J. S., Romero, I., Nava, M., & Huang, D. (2001). The role of language, parents, and peers in ethnic identity among adolescents in immigrant families. *Journal of Youth and Adolescence, 30*(2), 135–153. doi.org/10.1023/A:1010389607319

Pilcher, J. (2016). Names, bodies and identities. *Sociology, 50*(4), 764–779. doi:10.1179/nam.1983.31.4.245

Priven, D. (2008). Grievability of first language loss: Towards a reconceptualisation of European minority language education practices. *International Journal of Bilingual Education and Bilingualism, 11(*1), 95–106. doi.org/10.2167/beb414.0

Punzi, E. H. (2014). Freud's Jewish identity, circumcision, and the theory of castration anxiety: Problem or pride? *Mental Health, Religion and Culture, 17*(10), 967–976. doi.org/10.1080/13674676.2014.980721

Rizalar, S., Tural Buyuk, E., & Yildirim, N. (2017). Children's perspectives on the medical and cultural aspects of circumcision. *Iranian Journal of Pediatrics, 27*(2), e7561. https://ijp.tums.pub/en/articles/7561.html doi: 10.5812/ijp.7561

Russell, A. (2020). Black therapy matters blog. Retrieved from: www.blacktherapymatters.com/ 20 August 2020.

Şahin, F. U., Beyazova, U., & Akturk, A. (2003). Attitudes and practices regarding circumcision in Turkey. *Child: Care, Health and Development, 29*(4), 275–280. doi.org/10.1046/j.1365-2214.2003.00342.x

Said, E. W. (2003). *Orientalism*. Harmondswoth: Penguin.

Smith, F. D., Woo, M., & Austin, S. B. (2010). 'I didn't feel like any of those things were me': Results of a qualitative pilot study of race/ethnicity survey items with minority ethnic adolescents in the USA. *Ethnicity and Health, 15*(6), 621–638. doi.org/10.1080/13557858.2010.503872

Sue, D. W., & Sue, D. (2016). *Counseling the culturally diverse: Theory and practice,* 7th ed. Hoboken, NJ: Wiley.

Thomas, P. (2019). Neoliberalism: What it is and why it matters. In C. Jackson and R. Rizq (Eds.). *The industrialisation of care: Counselling, psychotherapy and the impact of IAPT* (pp. 1–12). Monmouth: PCCS Books.

Torgovnik, M. (1990). *Gone Primitive: Savage intellects, modern lives*. London: University of Chicago Press.

Tuckwell, G. (2002). *Racial identity, white counsellors and therapists*. Buckingham: Open University Press.

Tudor, K. (2018). *Psychotherapy: A critical examination*. Monmouth. PCCS Books.

Tuhiwai Smith, L. (2012). *Decolonising methodologies: Research and indigenous peoples,* 2nd ed. London: Zed books.

United States Census Bureau. (2012) News releases. Available at www.census.gov/newsroom/releases/archives/race/cb12-182.html

van Gennep, A. (1960). *The rites of passage*. London: Routledge & Kegan Paul.

Watters, E. (2010). *Crazy like us: The globalization of the western mind*. London: Constable & Robinson.

Yomtoob, D. (2014). Caught in code. In R. Boylorne & M. Orbe (Eds.). *Critical autoethnography. Intersecting cultural identities in everyday life* (pp. 144–158). Orange, CA: Left Coast Press.

Chapter 11

I refuse to choose

Culture, trans-culturalism and therapy

Sim Roy-Chowdhury

Summary

In this exploration of culture and trans-culturalism theoretical accounts are offered which are able to capture the complexity of the experience of migration. These accounts are considered within the context of a psychological therapy.

Introduction

I should suggest that an exploration of the meaning of culture and the promotion of an approach to psychotherapy that is sensitive to cultural difference is an act of subversion in the UK in 2021. The Brexit vote brought to the surface xenophobia and racism in Britain. Indeed far-right nationalism is on the rise in Europe, the US, India and around the world. A US president has been supported by the Ku Klux Klan, there is an Indian prime minister whose Citizenship Amendment Act seeks to deny Muslim people of Indian citizenship and in the UK a government that has adopted the policies of the far-right party, UKIP. It is a central tenet of these nationalistic movements that society is divided into us and them, with an entirely spurious homogeneity within each of these imagined groups. My interest in trans-culturalism, a propensity to locate oneself within more than one culture, across cultures, is a riposte to this far-right worldview.

Psychology and psychotherapy is situated within these nationalistic discourses and the profession of clinical psychology has had its own struggles to move its theoretical base and practice away from a Euro-American hegemony imposed upon people irrespective of their cultural referents. A disturbing level of cultural insensitivity within the profession has recently resurfaced in the enacting of a slave auction as evening entertainment at the annual conference for the Group of Trainers in Clinical Psychology (GTiCP) who lead the training programmes for clinical psychology. Patel et al. (2020) give voice to the outrage felt by therapists and among service users: 'Racism and complicity in racism is always wrong … Never entertainment' (p. 4). Writers including myself (Roy-Chowdhury, 2013) have argued that a change in practice amongst therapists must be accompanied by structural and systemic changes in the delivery and organisation of psychological therapy services, placing these services outside traditional settings, where 'therapy' is constructed and provided alongside, in partnership with members of local communities. Evidence of a pressing need for changes in theory, practice and structure is provided by a MIND survey (MIND, 2013) of users of Improving Access to Psychological Therapies (IAPT) services that found as few at 10% of people who identified themselves as coming from an ethnic minority background felt that their therapist had demonstrated an adequate level of cultural sensitivity, in contrast to 75% of therapists who believed their own practice to be culturally sensitive. Consequently, Khan (2020) argues that for 'people of colour' psychological therapies are not fit for purpose.

In Salman Rushdie's (1994) semi-autobiographical short story, to be found in *East West*, the author's alter ego settles in 1960s London with his family and his aya (nanny). His aya falls mysteriously ill, an illness with no physical causation, but rather, that she feels her heart 'roped by two different loves', being pulled East and West. Like the horses in the film, *The Misfits*, 'yanked this way by Clark Gable and that way by Montgomery Clift'. She returns to India; he stays in England and becomes a British citizen:

> the passport did, in many ways set me free … allowed me to make choices that were not the ones my father would have wished. But I, too, have ropes around my neck, I have them to this day, pulling me this way and that, East and West, the nooses tightening, commanding, choose, choose. I buck, I snort, I whinny, I rear, I kick. Ropes, I do not choose between you. Lassoes, lariats, I choose neither of you, and both. Do you hear? I refuse to choose.
>
> (p. 211)

This then is a chapter about culture, tranculturalism and therapy across cultures. It is also an exploration of the meaning of culture, particularly where an individual locates herself within more than one culture. For two such people working within a therapy context, how can we make sense of the numerous cultural influences evoked? I find in much of my work and writing that I emphasise the complex interplay of influences upon each individual subjectivity and encourage resistance against explanations that fix the individual within homogenising, reductive accounts. This is, no doubt, one expression of my own internal experience of cultural diversity, of a refusal to choose between two cultural identities.

For this particular scientist-practitioner, this then is also a personal account of my own struggles to understand the meaning and significance of culture in my own life and then to move from personal to professional understandings.

'Homesickness is not a real disease'

I left Calcutta, with my mother and brother, to join my father in Glasgow where he was studying medicine. At the tender age of 18 months, I have no recollection of the journey from my family home in Calcutta to my father's student flat in Glasgow. I do, however, have a powerful narrative for this transition passed on to me by my parents and my wider family in India. We left a comfortable middle-class life, populated by a large network of family members, and a rambling family home replete with servants and ayas, for a small, cold flat in Scotland. My parents left behind a comfortable life for a life of hardship and struggle in order that my father should establish himself as a doctor. The plan was that we would return to India but one position led to another for my father; my brother and I became settled in school, we moved to London and we settled in the UK. My parents had two clear trans-cultural policies in place for their two sons. The first was that we would speak English at home (although they would often talk to us in Bengali) in order to become proficient in our adopted language. The other that we would be steeped in our cultural heritage and, with this in mind, from the age of seven I spent large chunks of my childhood living in my second home in Calcutta. I grew up as a child adored by many adults: uncles, aunts, grandparents, etc. Each time I left the merry chaos of my family home, shared with my uncle and aunt, grandparents, cousin, to return to the cool reserve of England and our very English nuclear family, there were floods of tears, from children and adults alike. But of course there were compensations. I had great fun at primary school; the epithet that stuck to me at that time was that I was 'cheeky', in a semi-permanent state of irreverence, at any moment just a look or a remark away from laughter. It was not until I went to secondary school that I really encountered racism, although then I would not have thought of my experience as being defined by this grand word. This was the 1970s Britain of accelerating immigration, the Ugandian Asian crisis and Enoch Powell's inflammatory rhetoric. Despite great geopolitical shifts it was the everyday expression of prejudice in the sitcoms of the day that had the most immediate impact upon my life. Popular comedy shows such as *Love Thy Neighbour*, offered my classmates a complete lexicon of prejudice; people of colour were identified by such terms as wogs, sambos and nignogs. My barely conscious and wholly unoriginal response to this racism was to suppress expressions of my Indian cultural identity and to live my life as if I were a member of the indigenous English society. Such a choice between cultural referents had the additional advantage of providing me with a route-map through the landscape of a youthful rebellion against the preferences of my parents (my father, in particular). I came to adopt some of the prejudices that were inflicted upon me and gazed with a world-weary eye upon the illiberal constraints of my Bengali culture; the prohibition on sexual partners and cohabitation outside marriage and the preference for arranged marriages, I dismissed as archaic and anachronistic injunctions. Later, through my own personal psychotherapy, I searched for my own cultural voice, which was not wholly English or Indian, but both. My father's lengthy illness coincided with becoming a father myself, and both experiences afforded opportunities to reconcile my Indian heritage with my English context. However, these two cultures do not coexist harmoniously and there are often tensions between cultural narratives, most evident at times that I have had to make key life choices. I have written elsewhere of these struggles in relation to fatherhood and masculinity (Roy-Chowdhury, 2007). In that paper I follow the conventions of an academic article, with carefully referenced assertions, although, in essence, it is a tale of two cities, of a boy from Calcutta, trying to be a man in London.

Culture: what it is and what it is not

I give the autobiographical account in the preceding section not only to allow the reader to locate the authorial voice, to understand where I am coming from, as it were, but also as a starting point in the project to construct a theory of culture and the process of trans-culturalism. If we make the assumption that my experience is not unique and that others make equally finely contoured and idiosyncratic cultural transitions, how then can we construct an account of this phenomenon that captures its complexity and then apply this understanding to the context of a psychological therapy? First of all, the easy bit, what is it that culture is not? Culture is defined in the following way in a booklet issued to mark World Mental Health Day, 2007:

> Culture is the collective programming of the human mind that distinguishes the members of one human group from those of another. Culture in this sense is a system of collectively-held values.
>
> (World Federation for Mental Health, 2007)

Within the terms of this definition culture is a fixed, static set of characteristics attributable to a group of people who share a culture. One might, for example, take this definition to provide camouflage for various stereotyped assumptions and prejudices of the sort that German holiday-makers put their towels on the poolside sun-loungers first thing in the morning or that Indian men prefer their wives to look after the home. Such a static, de-contextualised, definition allows for little movement for people within a cultural location, all of whom are seen to share a common view of the world. The definition cannot accommodate the experience of trans-culturalism, where individuals position themselves uniquely and idiosyncratically to more than one set of cultural referents. We can see the pervasive influence of cultural referents even in the definitional preferences that can come to dominate within that culture. The WFMH definition posits that culture is 'programmed' into the individual mind, which draws our attention to the propensity for collectivist phenomena to be reinvented within the ambit of Western individualism. The Euro-American 21st-century predilection for computer metaphors to describe the human condition is also in evidence. The reader will have detected a dissatisfaction with such essentialist definitions. They do not seem to me to capture the complexity of the phenomenon that we observe; they certainly do not allow me to construct an account that would capture my own trajectory through culture. My preference is for Krause's (1998) ethnographic representations of culture. She makes use of the work of the anthropologist Geertz (1993) in defining culture as:

> A web of meaning rather than a series of patterns of behaviour and the anthropologist can study this web as she studies a collection of texts by straining 'to read over the shoulders of those to whom they properly belong … Societies like lives contain their own interpretations'.
>
> (Krause, 1998: 16, quoting Geertz, 1993: 452–453)

Hence, culture does not only make available to the individual a behavioural repertoire, but presents particular orientations toward behaviour, which provide contexts for understanding beliefs, motivations and emotions. An important aspect of the definition of culture that I am proposing is its interactional and contextually bound nature. Each individual is positioned uniquely in relation to the repertoires of meaning and behaviour available within a culture, and enacts this positioning in contextually specific ways. Culture is made and remade within each interaction and within each social context. Laird (1998, pp. 28–29) puts it in this way:

> culture is an individual and a social construction, a constantly evolving and changing set of meaning … it is always contextual, emergent, improvisational, transformational and political; above all it is a matter … of languaging, of discourse.

The contextually bound nature of cultural expression may seem to some readers a somewhat abstract idea; let me see if I can explain it from my experience. I have been to Calcutta to visit my family accompanied by two partners (on separate occasions, of course), who are English and had previously not known me in an Indian context. Each of those two people have remarked upon the transformation of the person whom they had thought that they each knew rather well into someone other than that person. This is more than my use of the Bengali language, a mysterious and wholly subliminal use of Indian movements and gestures but also a more profound way of being in the world. A perhaps trivial example is the huge delight that I would take in storytelling within my family. The smallest incident, which, within an English interactional context, would barely warrant a remark would be spun into the most elaborate of tales, a Joycean epic created from an encounter with a spider in the bathroom. In Mira Nair's film, the *Namesake*, Gogol rediscovers his Bengali heritage when his father dies. Living in New York, his American girlfriend, finds him, shaven headed, dressed in Indian clothes, surrounded by family, performing a ceremony for his dead father. She barely recognizes him and tries to return to him the identity that she knows and loves, by invoking plans for a holiday together as a solution to his sadness and a return to American values of romantic love and hedonism. He looks at her as if he does not understand what she has said and she starts to cry. Her tears move him to say, 'This isn't about you.' By this he means that she has stripped the communal and familial significance of mourning rituals of their cultural location and placed within the ambit of the primacy of the individual and of the couple relationship.

Doing culture in therapy

Let us turn now to these considerations within the context of a psychotherapy. ('At last', you may well say, dear reader.). The task that I have set for myself in this section is to take the theoretical issues, the ways of imagining culture, described in the preceding section and to look at the implications of the application of different perspectives within the therapy context. Within a book chapter of this length it is not possible to encompass all models of therapy. Hence, in acknowledgement of my dual professional identities, as clinical psychologist and systemic psychotherapist, I shall confine myself to therapy with families. I shall, of necessity, indicate which approach to culture I find more or less therapeutically helpful; though whilst fence-sitting is to be avoided, so too is pedagogy. This is not intended to be a guide to the right way of talking about culture in therapy. I am aided in my endeavour by an earlier co-written paper (Pakes and Roy-Chowdhury, 2007), which describes part of a qualitative research study. It is important to give credit where it is due: I supervised the research but Kirsty Pakes was the researcher. The aim of the study was to subject family therapy sessions to a discursive analysis in order to analyse the ways in which culture is evoked in therapy talk and the effects upon participants of these various ways of talking about therapy. One of our findings concerned the effects upon participants of the reification of culture. We found that:

> The discursive effects in the therapy of assumptions relating to a reified account of 'culture' are shown to constrain the conversation through the construction of artificial dichotomies and limited and troubled subject positions. These constraining discursive effects can be linked to reduced cultural sensitivity … because the complexity of 'culture' and peoples' positions in relation to 'culture' cannot be fully taken into account.
>
> (Pakes & Roy-Chowdhury, 2007, 281)

We discovered that where culture is talked into being as a homogeneous set of beliefs held by those who belong to that culture, this closes down the therapeutic space for people to express their own complex and perhaps contradictory positioning in relation to a variety of cultural influences that are created differently within different ecological niches. A conversational reification of culture (for example, in relation to family communication, marital choice, career decisions) does not capture the trajectory of cultural transition. Rather, only a more limiting acceptance or rejection of cultural norms is available to participants, redolent of Derrida's (1978) logic of 'binary oppositions'. A view of culture as a homogeneous set of beliefs and practices is not at all uncommon, and indeed one might even identify this as the dominant Euro-American narrative. Hence, unsurprisingly, we find thoughtful clinicians constructing culture within these terms within a therapy context. For example, Burnham and Harris (1996) offer an extended case example for a consideration of culture in therapy. Queenie Harris is the therapist working with a family of Chinese origin living in England. The session begins with the therapist asking whether one of their children follows the 'norm' of 'Chinese families' by sleeping with his parents. The father resists a monolithic view of culture by referring to his 'liberal' approach which allows the children freedom to make their own choices and resists an imposition of Chinese norms as an explanation for their son's behaviour. This attempt by the therapist to reify culture, as something that one either follows or does not, surfaces throughout the session and is resisted by the family. The family talk about the relationship between their two sons, which they do not, themselves, attribute to cultural influences. However, the therapist continues to place this relationship within the ambit of culturally prescribed attitudes and behaviour. She enquires whether the parents believe that one of their sons does not act like a 'Chinese brother' and whether his behaviour is 'normal in Chinese families'. The couple try gamely to resist this reification of culture using various conversational gambits. At one point they resist the proposition that Chinese culture is responsible for their sons' behaviour by universalising the relationship as something that takes place 'in all families, it's bound to, all children have sibling rivalry' (p. 21). As a psychotherapist, how then might one avoid giving voice to this cultural narrative that culture can be conceptualised as something homogeneous and consistent, to which one either adheres or one does not in relatively unproblematic ways? Falicov (2005), always worth turning to in relation to this question, points up the complexity of 'emotional transnationalism', where migrants feel the pull of the cultures, mediated often not by direct experience but by intergenerational stories, and respond to these resonances in idiosyncratic ways. She draws upon a piece of qualitative research by Stone et al. (2005) which examines family stories of American migrant families, to point up the sheer unpredictability of the process of acculturation. She suggests to the clinician that 'linear acculturation theories are becoming outdated' and that one should keep in mind that:

> In most families, continuity and change are happening side by side, in creative non-linear ways. Some family members may adhere to certain customs, such as home remedies, but the same members, or others, may oppose the arranged marriages favoured in the culture. … More than ever,

> we have to tell ourselves not to stereotype but to ask about values and preferences with respectful curiosity.
>
> (p. 403)

Krause (1998) suggests that the benefits to the therapist of learning more about the lives lived by others, through travel, friendships, art, literature, is not only that we may be better informed about the shape of other people's lives but also that we may learn more about what it is that we take for granted. Drawing upon the work of the anthropologist and philosopher, Bourdieu (1990), she refers to this taken for granted assumptive base as 'doxic' material. This is the socially constructed basis upon which we take up our place in the world: it is how we think of our subjectivity, agency, the relationship between self and others, family patterns, hierarchies and inter-relationships. This material feels natural to us and hence we are only ever partially aware of its existence. However, open, meaningful contact with the lives that others lead allows us glimpses of this doxic material and helps us, as clinicians, to develop a greater awareness of the assumptions that we make. In support of this proposition I give my own recent experience of reading wonderful novels by Bernadine Avaristo (2019), Tayari Jones (2018) and Kiley Reid (2019) and the insights offered within them into of the lives of black women in the USA and UK and their struggles against racism and prejudice.

I would like to close with two brief accounts of clinical work, which I offer, not at all as exemplars to others but rather in the spirit of shared thinking about therapy across cultures. The work with these two families differed in many ways that will become apparent but there is a commonality in the nature of their loss. Needless to say I have changed details in order to preserve anonymity.

Case example 1

A family, who had come to England as young children from Nigeria, were referred to my family therapy service by a psychiatrist. Ben is in his forties and has a diagnosis of paranoid schizophrenia. He has two sisters, Mary, a few years older than him and Freda, a few years younger. Ben came to England with his parents as a young child, while his sisters remained in Nigeria in the care of the extended family. Their father was taken ill and died suddenly in Nigeria during a trip to attend to family business in the country, and shortly afterwards, Mary and Freda joined their mother, Rose, and brother in England. Following Ben's release from prison for a drugs-related offence, family relationships disintegrated. He blamed his mother for losing his money in a business venture, and there were serious episodes of violence involving Ben, his mother and his younger sister. At the time of referral, the referrer expressed doubts that the family could be in the same room together, and suggested that a high level of family conflict had led to an increase in Ben's distress (seen as a 'decrease in mental health').

The family did come to a first appointment together. I assessed the family, and was alerted at this early stage to the significance of issues of cultural transition for the family. Within my service the psychotherapist offering therapy and the assessor can be two different people. I explained this fact to the family at the end of the session but the family requested that I work as their therapist, and said they would be prepared to wait until I became available to them. This was a request that they explained in terms of a hypothesis that I would be well-placed to understand their experience of cultural transition. It is worth lingering upon this request for a moment. Clearly the cultures that I have at my disposal differ significantly to cultural referents available to the family members. Rather, it seemed that they wanted to make use of a therapist who might understand the processes of migration, acculturation, intergenerational differences, and to see these as unique and individually differentiated events. One might suppose that they wanted a therapist who had himself experienced the complexity of cultural transition, and the particular insight that one is afforded to the aspects of a culture that one takes for granted, one's doxic material.

The family therapy sessions that followed included various family subsystems at various times, as levels of potential conflict and violence were high in the early sessions. A key aspect of the work was to work on the bereavement that the siblings suffered as children when their father died. This grief had never been allowed expression by their mother as she felt herself too emotionally overwhelmed to deal with the profound loss, without risking a 'breakdown' herself. The family script was to throw themselves into activities and not to talk of their father. The money that Ben had left with his mother when he went to prison, and which she had lost in the family business, began to be seen for its symbolic significance, as a proxy for loss and the grief that could not be expressed. As we talked, cultural influences upon each of them were referenced many times, implicitly and explicitly. They often talked about how an experience might be constructed 'back home' or by 'the family'. The three siblings talked about culturally congruent rituals in relation to their father's illness and subsequent death and the attitudes that people 'at home' would have to the roles of boys and girls, men and women. We explored their positioning in relation to British and Nigerian culture, and discovered differences between each of them and anger at their mother for holding fast to attitudes and practices that were, they asserted, in tune with the family but that they struggled to accommodate within their lives in England. She, on the other hand, said things to them that they had never heard, of her devastation at losing her beloved husband, her feelings of loss and utter bewilderment on her own in this strange land, with three children looking to her for guidance. When she took these actions that she hoped would be in their best interests, such as bringing Nigerian 'elders' into their home to discipline them, they began to realise that she was doing the best that she could. We dealt with the violence in difficult sessions. Ben was 'shocked' to hear what his actions had done to the sister who had, until then, looked up to her older brother. One cannot heal these wounds in a session or two but the first steps toward reparation were taken as she heard him speak of his deep sorrow and shame at his actions. Here too culture surfaced in his account of masculinity and in the place within the family afforded to the eldest son. When an aspect of their lives was constructed as holding within it a cultural meaning, I might enquire where each of them might position themselves and each other within these webs of meaning. I might also enquire how the similarities and differences emerged in their relationships, in their interactions with each other and others in their lives. These proved to be fruitful avenues for exploration. The strength and resilience of women within the family was pieced together as a narrative supported by two sets of cultural influences, and enacted with Mary and Freda's British-born husbands. A place was found for Ben which accommodated the twin sets of influences upon this family, where for the first time he felt that he had something of value that he could offer the rest of the family. There were times that I misread the place of culture as a strand within the thread of the therapy talk. But as there were also many more occasions that my prompts found a resonance with them they were able to forgive me my lapses. The family have discovered new ways of being a family and of being both British and Nigerian. They have shown enormous generosity toward each other, and have walked some way along a path of forgiveness.

Case example 2

I have chosen my work with this family in order to explore the premise that a cultural similarity between therapist and therapees may be offered as a solution to the problems encountered in therapy by 'people of colour' (Khan, 2020).

Sanjay and his two brothers and two sisters, all older than him, were born in England, his mother Jaya was born in India. The whole family lived in the UK and both mother and youngest son were referred to my service following the death of Apu, Jaya's husband, Sanjay's father. At the heart of their problems with anxiety and intense sadness was a process of grieving for Apu that was complicated by the narrative among their other children that Apu had shown a preference for Sanjay in his will, which was confirmation to them that he was his father's favourite child. As one would expect, Sanjay's siblings took varied and unique positions in relation to this narrative; however, it took such a strong hold within the family that Sanjay felt isolated from his siblings whose anger and hurt left him feeling abandoned at such a difficult time. For his mother it was her worst nightmare that, having lost her beloved husband, it felt as if her family was breaking up.

During the course of the therapy I listened to Jaya and Sanjay's desperate sadness at their loss of Apu. I talked with them about their relationship with each other with Apu and wider sibling and parental relationships. Sanjay was the only unmarried sibling with no other couple relationship ties when his father died and this was given as the reason that he moved into his parents' home in order to support his mother. He had indeed had a close relationship with his father and, because of this relationship and his experience in finance, Sanjay was left by his father the responsibility of selling a family home that his parents still owned in India. Due at least in part to my awareness of the culturally influenced beliefs that can be found in Indian families I asked questions about how this assignment of responsibilities had been understood by other family members. I knew from experience that there is often an expectation that the oldest child takes a more dominant position in dealing with such matters rather than, as in this family, the youngest. Hence I could ask questions about this from the perspective of other family members, although I should say that I felt that these questions, these invitations to see through the eyes of other family members, only had the impact that they did because I had tried so hard to understand the difficulties that they faced from their perspectives. Over the course of the therapy this greater understanding of the views taken by others within the family led to their decision to end the sessions. At the final session Sanjay remarked that their relationships felt 'almost normal'.

Hence this therapeutic encounter supports the hypothesis that shared cultural referents can be helpful. Having said this I recall an occasion where Jaya questioned the presuppositions that may have informed my questions, and indeed perhaps in doing so drew upon the culturally influenced expectation of a respect for elders to be found within Indian families. She drew my attention to the peculiar idiosyncrasies of relationships within her family. Her eldest son was often away due to his work and she suggested that he was a rather distant, disengaged figure, which therefore moderated the view held by the family of his power and authority. This particular interaction strikes me as a reminder that for the therapist to have access to culturally influenced discourses might be helpful, and yet there is still the risk of making assumptions; hence it is just as important as in therapies where there are cultural differences for the therapist to question her own beliefs and to ask about the lives of others in a tentative manner. In this specific instance of a correction by Jaya of the application of a culturally influenced narrative to her family it was important for me as the therapist to offer my thoughts and questions in a provisional manner and to accept the correction provided by Jaya for she is, after all, the expert, when it comes to her own family. It also allowed me to take a deferential position (not that I would have theorised it in this way in the moment by moment interactions that took place) which was in tune with a respect for one's elders.

A conclusion

In writing this piece, I have been aware that I have run the risk of making the work of colleagues harder not easier. Writers who tackle this subject are right to worry about deskilling the reader, in providing a prescription for cross-cultural practice, to which fellow clinicians must adhere. The striking of this careful balance where culture is available as a construct that can open up, rather than close down, spaces for people in making sense of their lives may come to be seen as requiring enormous skill of the clinician. In outlining the two very different clinical encounters I have sought to avoid this by drawing upon an approach to therapy that puts a concern with fostering a strong therapeutic relationship (Roy-Chowdhury, 2015) and the taking of a non-expert position (Anderson and Goolishian, 1992) at the core of this endeavour. My conclusion rejoices in the simplicity of the interventions available to the psychotherapist in prompting the emergence of stories of culture. During my own lengthy psychotherapy, on occasion, following an account that I might give of an aspect of my life, my therapist would pause, reflect and enquire, 'I wonder if there might be a cultural dimension to this?' That would be all. I would be free to either take up this thought, or, as the suggestion was made with such humility, to reject it. I realise that I am at risk of idealising these therapeutic encounters but I do not recall a time that I felt this simple question to be unhelpful.

References

Anderson, H., & Goolishian, H. (1992). The client is the expert: A not-knowing approach to therapy. In *Therapy as social construction* (pp. 25–39). London: Sage.

Avaristo, B. (2019). *Girl, woman, other.* London: Penguin Random House UK.

Bourdieu, P. (1990). *The logic of practice.* Stanford, CA: Stanford University Press.

Burnham, J., & Harris, Q. (1996). Emerging ethnicity: A tale of three cultures. In K. N. Dwivedi & P. V. Varma (Eds.). *Meeting the needs of minority children* (pp. 160–174). London: Jessica Kingsley.

Derrida, J. (1978). *Writing and difference.* Chicago, IL: University of Chicago Press.

Falicov, C. J. (2005). Emotional transnationalism and family identities. *Family Process, 44,* 399–406.

Geertz, C. (1993 [1973]). Thick description: Toward an interpretive theory of culture. In C. Geertz (Ed.). *The interpretation of cultures* (pp. 3–32). London: Fontana.

Jones, T. (2018). *An American marriage.* London: Oneworld Publications.

Khan, C. (2020). Therapy has a long history of oppression. *The Guardian,* 12 July, 4–5.

Krause, I. B. (1998). *Therapy across culture* (1st ed.). London: Sage.

Laird, J. (1998). Theorizing culture: Narrative ideas and practice principles. In M. McGoldrick (Ed.). *Revisioning family therapy: Race, culture and gender in clinical practice* (pp. 20–36). New York: Guilford Press.

MIND (2013). *We still need to talk: A report on access to talking therapies.* London: MIND.

Pakes, K., & Roy-Chowdhury, S. (2007). Culturally sensitive therapy? Examining the practice of crosscultural family therapy. *Journal of Family Therapy, 29,* 267–283.

Patel. N. (2020). Racism is not entertainment. Letter published in *Clinical Psychology Forum,* 326, 2–5.

Reid, K. (2019). *Such a fun age.* London: Bloomsbury.

Roy-Chowdhury, S. (2008). Fatherhood and masculinity. *Context, 96,* 3–7.

Roy-Chowdhury, S. (2013), How can an IAPT service increase its cultural sensitivity? *Clinical Psychology Forum, 241,* 45–50.

Roy-Chowdhury, S. (2015). Why does a systemic psychotherapy 'work'? In M. O'Reilly & J. N. Lester (Eds.). *The Palgrave handbook of child mental health* (pp. 194–216). Basingstoke: Palgrave Macmillan.

Rushdie, S. (1994). *East, West,* 1st ed. London: Jonathan Cape.

Stone, E., Gomez, E., Hotzoglou, D., & Lipnitsky, J. Y. (2005). Transnationalism as a motif in family stories. *Family Process, 44*, 381–398.

World Federation for Mental Health (2007) *Mental health in a changing world: The impact of culture and diversity.* www.encontrarse.pt/wp-content/uploads/2016/12/docs_wfmh2007.pdf

Chapter 12

Echo to authenticity

Exploring identity in an age of privilege and supremacy

Dwight Turner

Summary

Ideas of how identity forms have a long tradition within the worlds of psychology and psychotherapy. What is less understood though is how identity is challenged when we are a minority having to negotiate a world not of one's own gender, race, or culture. Through the client example of a psychology student of colour, and using intersectionality theory, this chapter explores how the identity as the other fluctuates when it encounters cultural, racial or gendered privilege and supremacy, recognising some of the survival techniques used by the other to survive said experience, together with the cost to one's own mental health.

Introduction

Several years ago, a student psychotherapist, who was also a client of mine, told me the following story. They explained that they recently had to attend a workshop on difference and diversity as part of the third year of a four-year post-graduate course in Counselling and Psychotherapy. During this two-hour lecture, the discussion inevitably moved on to race and difference. Having not spoken much during lectures for the previous two years, the student felt that this was the first opportunity she might have to say all the things she had wanted. So, when her opportunity came, she spoke of her pain at being an outsider, her fear as a woman of colour in a world that is mainly white and her sense of not feeling seen by her peers.

Within a few minutes of her speaking up, another participant, a white woman, burst into tears, expressing both anger and sadness at the experience and the words uttered by my client. At this point in the proceedings, the other students in the cohort, who were mainly white, then sided with the other white, female, student, comforting her, and making her feel safe, whilst leaving my client on her own, feeling silenced and unseen, just as she had expressed moments earlier in her monologue to the group. The facilitator did nothing to change the situation.

This type of interaction, and these types of stories, are all too familiar in training courses it appears. Where there is a growing 'pseudo-comfort' with acknowledging diversity within trainings, it also appears that we are, as psychologists and psychotherapists, intellectually unprepared for the unconscious challenges that working with difference and diversity bring with it. The idea that workshops on these topics should be a tokenistic add-on at the side of a training course fails to truly explore the problem of inequality, or to demystify its cultural spectre. It could be argued that this performative provision of diversity workshops has done little more than to maintain the cultural status quo, instead of revealing its fullest supremacist aspects. For example, as Bhopal (2018) recognises in her work, equality politics has predominantly benefited one group, that being white, middle-class, heterosexual women, both in the world of academia and wider society. She also notes that the levels of inequality for other groups, LGBTQ, BAME, disabled people, etc. have not changed that much in comparison.

A perfect example of this comes from a BBC story exploring the disparity in pay for academics. In their study they noted that white women were paid 15% less than white men, whereas Asian women (22%) and black women (39%) were paid considerably lower rates accordingly (Croxford, 2018). The importance of studies like this is to highlight the varying layers of oppression endured by those seen as different, as if there would not be individuals who might straddle both positions, and therefore have to deal with multiple layers of oppression within these, and therefore other, organisations and society. Bringing this more nuanced way of working with diversity to our trainings and practice so they become safer spaces to explore the dangerous and challenging aspects of sameness and otherness, thereby allowing students and practitioners alike to feel a greater sense of recognition and acceptance, is an essential component in the work. This chapter therefore explores just how a more intersectional approach to identity, together with an exploration of how privilege co-creates identity, therefore redefines our understanding of difference and diversity.

The problem of difference and identity

Stories like this one from the student are not uncommon within psychology and psychotherapy courses. Training courses often take a decidedly tokenistic approach to the exploration of issues around difference and diversity. For many students this absence then compounds an already prevalent sense of feeling unseen within their own training, and in effect within their future trades. Whilst issues of the absence of all types of difference have been addressed in many arenas, what is often not recognised is the psychological damage caused by such an experience. The lack of mirroring, the paucity of trainers of difference, be they of colour, women or LGBTQ, often brings with it for students from one or a multiple of these backgrounds a sense that they are invisible, that they do not matter or that they do not feel they exist at all.

The psychological damage here should not be understated. Whereas Lacan (2003) saw mirroring for a child through the loving gaze of its mother as a crucial stage of egoic development, there is a popular misconception that once we reach the age of maturity we no longer need such mirroring, or such guidance. This is an incredibly flawed belief. Throughout life we find ourselves in certain groups where we are with people who are *like us*, before leaving them and finding other groups who are the same. These could be groups of Goths, working mothers, academics or those who Cosplay at conventions. They could also be British expats living abroad in Spain, protestors of the Far Right or Antifa in the United States of America, or the Yellow Jackets protesting on the streets of Paris during the 2019 riots. That need to fit in, that need to be a part of something, allows us to feel safe, to feel recognised and accepted. It allows us to feel seen and have a sense of who we are.

Although a term much criticised politically currently, the ideas that formed the origins of the political correctness movement were actually designed to encourage discussions between feminists, where they could, amongst many other aspects, formulate ideas and perspectives that maybe sat outside the patriarchal political narratives of the time (Digby, 1992). These spaces therefore allowed women to be met by women. To be mirrored, to be witness and to know who they were in relation to their peers. Yet this is an aspect of the experience of the other which is often ignored, or even worse denigrated; the need for safe spaces for the other, or for a sense they are included in the general narratives within their training courses.

The danger is that training spaces have therefore become spaces dominated by the presence of central forces who then dominate the narrative and are reluctant to relinquish any of this territory to the other, out of a fear of having their power usurped. Tokenism maintains this positioning whereby the other is given a role or a seat at the top tables, but there is no autonomy, no will to make the changes they are quite capable of making. Others include bootstrapping, where the other is encouraged to believe they have the same opportunities as those of privilege, and that to succeed they only have to do the same as those who sit more centrally.

That there is an element of narcissism in this perspective is obvious (Benjamin, 1998). An idea which within psychotherapy has been discussed by authors such as Freud, Lacan and Jung, narcissism simply put involves the idea that one forms an egoic identity through the mirrored presence and reflection of our primary caregivers (Cratsley, 2015; Homer, 2007; Morrison, 1986). Narcissism here therefore involves the idea that, without an other to perform this function, we struggle to have a true sense of who we are. Yet, within these spaces, within this narcissistic need to be acknowledged, there is often the marginalisation of the other.

So, for the other on training courses, often the only route out of not being seen, and surviving on these courses where privilege reigns supreme, is by adopting the position of the echo to narcissus. The problem with this position is the inauthenticity that it can create within the other. An idea posited by Spivak (1993), the sense that in order to survive in non-other environments one has to adapt to ways of being not of one's own culture, gender or sexuality is not a new one. One of the most interesting examples I ever encountered was of a student who for the four-year duration of her counselling course had hidden her hearing disability in order to not be marked out as different, and therefore marginalised, because she might have needed additional support.

To explore this further, Ovid's (2015) original myth is therefore useful. From the book *Metamorphoses*, when Echo first met Narcissus she instantly fell for him but would not let herself be seen by him. Hiding in bushes nearby him, she then took to repeating as best as she could each phrase that he uttered, often only reflecting back to him aspects of his utterances. This led to Narcissus becoming enraged with this unseen voice, so much so that he berates her, forcing her to leave him alone. One means of surviving within environments not one's own is to be compliant, to conform with a means of being that keeps the majority feeling comfortable. To be a psychological echo of those in the position of power.

One of the reasons for this is the power dynamic is emergent from learning or teaching from texts by male, white, middle-class, heterosexual, authors, thereby marginalising any voices of the other accordingly. This experience is then internalised by the other, leading to an unconscious leaning towards that same normative narrative in how they present, be it literally or in their work. For example, during a seminar I ran on exploring difference in research, a group of predominantly white female students were asked to name three famous psychotherapists and three therapists that they admire. In this unscientific exercise, over 70% of the therapists named were white men, a statistic which when reflected to the students themselves led to a vigorous debate as to which theorists they had been taught, who they were drawn towards, and why. Even though this example is emergent out of a psychotherapy training, this is in no way limited to our fields within the helping professions. We are all, to varying degrees, indoctrinated into the system of white, middle to upper class, heteronormative, supremacy, no matter how we self-identify as the other in the rest of our lives.

Returning to the student example, then, one aspect that puzzled me in our work was the idea of survival. On exploring this with her, we realised that she had learnt to 'fit in'; to not be too loud, wear anything too ethnic, to not appear too black. The student recognised that this fear of being seen as too much the other was based upon a sense that, were she deemed as such, she would be excluded from her course, leading to months of anxiety and shuttling between trying to be more authentic within her training against being that which she felt her tutors needed her to be. During a deeper psychological discussion about this experience, the student also recognised that to inhabit the position of the echo also meant that she would have to unconsciously destroy that which made her uniquely different or the other; the message to not be too black, or too ethnic. This contrasted with the positioning of herself as the other, and the psychological isolation that this could engender within her, versus or in addition to any possible sense of psychological self-destruction brought about by a sense that she no longer existed in relation to her peers or her course. This shuttling between positioning oneself as the other or the echo, or between authenticity and inauthenticity, thereby leads to increased psychological distress over time.

These types of experiences are not uncommon aspects of the other's experience of being in a world that is not their own, and stories of this type are not uncommon. From women who feel they have to hide aspects of their femininity when in groups of men at work, to the lesbian couple fearful of holding hands in public, the fear of at best some type of micro-aggression, at worst overt physical and verbal abuse, sits central to those who are deemed different by the subject.

Echoism therefore becomes a means of survival for the other when faced with the narcissism of those with power. This therefore means that those with power get to dictate the narratives of the courses they teach upon, unchallenged by the other, because it has more often than not had to ingratiate itself within the ranks of those of privilege. The identity of the other, when they encounter that which is deemed normative, is therefore either seduced into the position of the echo, or is exiled to the position of the outsider. Raising awareness of the potential for psychological harm towards the other when entering a space not of their own is therefore hugely important for the other to feel included. This though can only occur in relation to a deeper understanding of just what identity is, and how it is formed. This is particularly important given the varying layers of difference and otherness which construct our identity, with an intersectional understanding of this construction being central to our understanding of this identity formation.

An intersectional identity

In her work on power in relation to the other, Haug (2008) explores the idea that knowledge is governed from a central position, and that the other is identified from this centralised point. This is important to recognise when we consider who is deemed to be the other, and who is not. Within the patriarchal political structures, for example, those who are deemed different are cared for through current legislation, such as the Equality Act 2010 where the protected characteristics are age, disability, gender reassignment, marriage and civil partnership, pregnancy and maternity, race, religion or belief, sex, and sexual orientation. That these protected characteristics have had to be fought for over a number of years shows their undeniable importance, but the idea that difference is only limited to those who identify as the other dependent upon nine politically defined characteristics is extremely problematic. Also troubling is the idea that these characteristics can often only be considered individually, especially when we ask questions such as what happens when an individual is discriminated against because of their age as well as their religion or their beliefs? These are two different protected characteristics, and how they are experienced will vary accordingly.

Identity and experiences as the other are therefore not limited to one of these characteristics. As Crenshaw (Carastathis, 2014) discusses, in her development of an intersectional approach to understanding difference, the experiences of women of colour were divided by both race and gender, and the legislation of the time struggled to incorporate both aspects of identity fully. What this meant was that women of colour had to choose the form of oppression they were experiencing based upon the limits of their legal system. So, although identity is multifaceted, the problem of understanding experiences of difference are compounded by the varying layers of said same differences. This is where the ideas of intersectionality then become important.

The origins of intersectionality though are open to debate. As Hill Collins and Bilge discuss, it is generally accepted that the debate around intersectionality emerged out of the United States in the 1960s and 1970s, where 'the intellectual production and activism of black women, Chicanas, Asian-American women, and Native American women were not derivative of the so-called second-wave white feminism but were original in their own right' (2016, 65). Within the African American community in the 1970s though, intersectionality found its more academic voice. For example, one of its pioneers, Kimberle Crenshaw, developed intersectionality as a means of working on a deeper level with issues of difference and otherness, moving beyond even this triangular means of seeing difference, and beginning to deepen its meaning dependent upon the composite of forms of identity that we all hold at any given time in our lives (Cho et al., 2013). Her work on developing a theory to explore these intersectional ways of seeing equality recognised that we all often suffer from a multiple, intersecting layers of oppression as we go about our day-to-day existence.

Broadening this approach further though, there have subsequently been many papers that have taken an intersectional approach to understanding difference. For example, this is a position explored in Mereish's wonderful (2012) paper on the intersecting experiences of prejudice when individuals hold a racial difference and a disability, whilst Brooks (2010) uses intersectionality to combine feminist thinking and the transpersonal in exploring spiritual experiences of women. Other interesting papers include Drazdowski's (2016) paper on the varying intersecting layers of discrimination experienced by LGBTQ persons of colour within their community.

The importance of an intersectional approach should not be underestimated. What an understanding of an intersectional difference and diversity does is to remove the power of identification away from the subject, returning it to the other. It also allows the other to experience their identity in their totality, allowing those multiple layers of otherness to then be experienced by the other; their gender, the sexual orientation, their race, culture, religion, their age, their profession. The importance of a totality of identity is relevant as identity is multifaced by its very nature, with all these sections of identity holding varying aspects of otherness or the individual or the collective group.

For example, for the female student of colour on her course, the idea that her only form of difference was that of gender then led to a marginalisation of her racial difference. It also meant the separation or negation of other more unconscious forms of difference; her possible class difference, the fact she was the daughter of immigrants and therefore seen as non-European, how her age might have played a part given the cultural predilection towards youth, or even any factors around her level of education when compared to that of her peers. These multiple aspects of identity will also make up aspects of who students are on their courses, meaning their difference will always be in the room with their peers, and with their future clients. To avoid them, or to pigeonhole difference into one of the few politically acceptable categories, then risks causing students additional psychological harm.

Intersectionality as a concept though is designed to more than just recognise the absence of non-white, heteronormative, examples of exclusion. What it does is to recognise that power dynamics are varied, that they are always present in interactions with the other, and that without a more nuanced understanding of power what we are left with are persons who will inevitably feel excluded through the inability of their training courses to recognise that their struggles might be different, but they might be real. The drive towards normativity that has long since influenced the helping professions is also a drive towards mirroring the exclusion of minorities that we witness daily in the external world. So, only through an intersectional approach to diversity politics can we even approach such an ideal of total inclusion, where by staying with the complex layering of power and difference we can even dare to approach the layers of inclusion necessary to avoid leaving minorities feeling marginalised within these same arenas where they are supposed to feel safest.

Privilege and identity

Ideas of privilege also need to be taken into consideration when we talk of identity, as this is an aspect of difference and sameness that is often overlooked when we enter the world of identity politics. Discussions of privilege often present this facet of identity as something negative and normally merged with power, therefore providing one's identity not only with its identification as other, but also as superior. For example, feminism has long ago identified the position of patriarchy as one of privilege, a positioning that left the woman as the other, not identified as herself, but in relation to that which was seen as the absolute, man (Beauvoir, 2010). Studies into just how long this process has endured for have presented varying perspectives, but one of the most interesting is emergent out of the work of Biewen and Headlee (2018) whose set of academic podcasts suggest that patriarchy is no more than 10,000 years old.

Another common form of privilege is whiteness. A social construct, as Appiah (2016) noted, whiteness needed its converse other, blackness, to exist, thereby binding their identities together. This is an area of interest again for Biewen (2017) whose series of podcasts considered the theoretical, scientific and religious creation of whiteness, its many varied aspects regularly presented as different, and better, stronger, more intelligent or more civilised than whiteness.

The worlds of psychology and psychotherapy have long failed to acknowledge their own complicity in maintaining these structures in the pathologising of behavioural or natural characteristics. For example, the sexist overuse of the diagnosis of hysteria against women from the early days of psychoanalysis has long been seen as a patriarchal attempt to demarcate and contain the behaviours of women (Kristeva, 1982). Simultaneously, within the world of psychiatry and psychology, homosexuality was long pathologised as an abnormal set of behaviours. In fact, the move to outlaw conversion therapy, a type of therapy designed to cure homosexuality and designed on either religious lines, or those derived from the 12 steps model for addictions, was only outlawed by the BACP, the BPS and numerous other therapeutic organisations in 2015 (Various, 2017). The fact that it has taken the worlds of psychology and psychotherapy so long to come to this agreement, and that Stonewall, the charity behind this Memorandum of Understanding, has had to work this hard to outlaw practices that have been seen as barbaric for decades, if not longer, is quite revealing. For example, it shows how entrenched heteronormative views on sexuality are within society, with homosexuality being pathologised, or with students feeling bullied, victimised or unseen upon many psychotherapy training courses until quite recently (Somerville, 2015).

To understand privilege on a deeper level though, the first thing to recognise is that it is problematic to automatically link privilege, power and supremacy together. Whilst those who hold the privilege of whiteness may well hold a sense of power over the identity of the other, this does not necessarily mean they automatically have a sense of superiority over them. These views also fail to recognise that when we combine privilege with power, and when it does become supremacy over the other, what we actually have is a type of narcissism which negates the identity of the other.

A perfect example arises in Lacan's idea of the child identifying itself in the mirrored gaze of the mother, when linked to the narcissistic omnipotent fantasy of the child, then there is a narcissistically imagined sense of superiority over the mother (Lacan, 2003). Hence narcissism, and supremacy, are therefore separate to privilege. Whilst a child who then struggles to recognise their mother's own identity as separate to them, or a child who has too much power over their parental caregivers, might grow up with a sense of superiority over others, any sense of known or unknown privilege may or may not be present. The child might have been born white, or have been born into a family with wealth, or be born male, but this does not necessarily mean that the child is aware of its privilege. What will develop over time though is the child's awareness of the levels of their cultural, gendered or heteronormative privilege, aspects of their identity reinforced by their parents, culture, society.

The issue of privilege is also not always a negative one, as I stated. Edward Said argued that the intellectual as the other has a specific role to play in identifying and offering an exploration of culture from the outside (Said, 1993). It is a position held by philosophers, for example, and also by musicians. For example, before David Bowie came out as gay back in the late 1960s in the music magazine *Melody Maker*, homosexuality was as much a hidden factor within the music industry as it was in wider society, thereby heralding a cultural change of perspective (Glen, 2012).

Privileges, and how they inform our intersectional identities, are also far more complex than the legally protected characteristics we are all aware of. At any given time, we might hold a number of different forms of privilege, be it being valued for our youth, being an academic or being born in Europe. They are also not static; the privilege of youth must give way to the increasing otherness of middle age and the invisibility of retirement age. We can earn them, not be aware of them, or lose them, dependent upon where we are, what we are doing, and the environment we are within at any moment of any day. Thus, this complex, constantly moving, aspect of our identity is not fixed; for example, who the reader is at home will be different to who they are when they enter their workplace, to when they walk through a less/more affluent area of their town, to when they are with or separate from people from their own gender, class, race, social strata, sexual minority. We are constantly negotiating aspects of privilege and otherness, and the varying aspects of power and powerlessness these entail, hundreds of times per day.

This was particularly important when working with the student. Originally, she saw herself as powerless to change things for herself on her course out of a fear of being judged as too much, or too black. Our work, though, assisted her in recognising that there was power in her privileged position as a woman of colour, who was studying at a high level, had already achieved a lot on her career, was living in Europe and who was heterosexual. She had money, a home and a sense of worth that many others of her peers had yet to achieve. These aspects of privilege, or power, originally projected outwards onto her course, and her peers, when returned to her helped her to in this instance find her voice in that room, enabling her to speak up about her experiences as the other.

Supremacy and shame

As already discussed, privilege comes in many forms, yet ideas of how privilege becomes supremacy differ. For writers such as Bhopal (2018) the idea of privilege is merged together with supremacy, as if one cannot have one without the other. This is a position echoed by Andrews (2018) in his work on the repositioning of black nationalism as an important discourse within the United Kingdom, or from Memmi's (1974) work on the inherent layered privilege of the French against those they colonised. Whilst all these perspectives speak of an inherent privilege that lies within the position of whiteness or the coloniser, as I have previously stated this conflation of privilege with supremacy is actually problematic.

An example of this problem emerges out of boarding school system. Originally constructed by the Ancient Greeks in order to ascertain who was right to lead their armies into war, the environment of the boarding school idea was so constructed to keep the strong and shed the weak (Duffell, 2014). An education system that then crafts those who will lead became a system which has lasted thousands of years, and is revered across the world, both by those within the said system, as much as by the rest of us led by those raised within it. It is in this instance harnessed, created and moulded as a means of being to be, to aspire towards, to be envious of and to desire to be with.

Alternatively, this system of cultural measurement, and supremacy is also used in the creation of the different genders. As Gilligan (1982) suggests in her ideas from a more psychotherapeutic perspective, when we come in to life, we are immediately subjected to a form of Binary Splitting, where from the variety of qualities and ways of being sitting in the collective unconscious, some are separated into masculine and feminine, and then good and bad, by men over women. It is important to recognise therefore that these theories of demarcation at their cores discuss the systemic creation of the gendered other. So, we already have two examples where identity is manipulated, where aspects of our own self are culturally harnessed, be it positively or negatively, for a culture to develop and maintain its dominion over the other.

The problem with these ideas though is that they work from a gendered, cultural or racial perspective. Yet, this process does not end with the separation of these groupings. This is a process that repeats itself, over and over, in the splitting of childhood groups by anything from the colour of a child's hair to the fact a peer is too thin, too big or too tall. Alternatively, as Piaget and Weil (1951) discuss in their work, children go through stages in their encounter with difference; for example, up until the age of seven years old, children move from a position of primary narcissism, where there is no other and where the other is not recognised as anything other than aspect of themselves; to one where they start to recognise the other and can with assistance relate to the other; to one where they can experience shame about their own cultural, or gendered, group, and have empathy for the other.

Much of this co-creation of identity is mitigated by the responses of family, culture and the wider social environment, so for those children who struggle with encounters with difference, often their fear is not managed. It is not contained, held, discussed or normalised, aspects that would be conducted with any other emotion, in any other situation, echoing the work of Bion (1985).

This lack of containment of course inevitably leads to an inability to handle encounters with the other. For example, Di Angelo's (2011) work around White Fragility suggests that, when confronted with issues around race, white people struggle with the psychological impact of such discussions upon their own racial identity. Yet, whilst this is an important aspect to consider, the issue of fragility, or the stress of the said majority or subject, is not just limited to the arena of race and whiteness. From a more patriarchal position, the idea of male fragility in the constant question of what is a man, how to be a man, and the feelings of men that they are being diminished in the face of feminism, are also important to notice as aspects of male fragility as this binary process repairs itself. A more modern-day version of this is the #notallmen hashtag raised in direct contradiction to the #metoo hashtag, and its important movement to raise the abuses of the gendered other by numerous men worldwide.

As discussed, we all hold some type of privilege, be it because of our sexual orientation, being male, racial, able-bodied or any other type of privilege, and that these types of privileges form a large part of our identities, with some changing over time, some being inherited, some being obtained through the course of one's life whilst simultaneously others are lost. This identity though is always fragile, no matter the form that it takes, as identity is fluid and constantly changing. The encounter with the other is one means that this identity is challenged. One of the means of countering this challenge to the fragility of identity is by taking a position of power over the other, whilst re-entrenching one's position, and therefore one's identity in relation to the other. Psychologically, privilege and the inability to handle the stress of the presence of the other, is the ego's attempts to control the presence of the shadow. The psychological defence against encounters with the other is therefore no different to the psychological defence of a counselling or psychotherapy client when they enter therapy. Both involve a potential encounter with difference, be it external or internal. This is where, from a Lacanian perspective, the internalised sense of superiority then emerges (Lacan, 2003).

Supremacy is therefore more than just patriarchal, cultural, sexual orientation or racial privilege in addition to power. It has evolved to become something far more systemic, to the extent that it permeates all our identities in some fashion. From the simple need for students on psychotherapy and psychology courses to compete with one another, to more overt undermining of colleagues that often occurs within the helping professions. This of course is nothing but a mirror of the need for society and its inhabitants to present themselves as superior, from the competitiveness of sports, the comparisons with one's neighbours because they have a better car, house or eat vegan food, comparison and competitiveness hold many of the aspects of supremacy that we are all driven to aspire towards. We are all pulled towards the black hole of supremacy in some fashion.

Other examples include the political drive to have migrants fit into a British way of life, which not only privileges this one way of life, but also holds within its makeup the implied belief that Britishness is superior to those cultural structures held by said immigrant. A perfect example is when Margaret Thatcher commissioned a report into the causes of the Brixton Riots which shook the country in the 1980s; one of the most unsurprising aspects they discovered was that their previous comfort in the supposed assimilation of those from the former colonies had not occurred at all (BBC, 2014). This is the cost of believing in the supremacy of one culture over another, or of forcing one culture to give up its identity in service to the subject culture. What it does is repress that which is true to its nature, until it emerges, often suddenly, often necessarily reactively, to remind the subject that it exists, that it has not gone away at all.

Returning to the student example, the student was from a Black British background, her parents being of Caribbean origin. During one session she told me a story about her father, who had travelled to the United Kingdom as part of the Windrush Generation of the late 1950s. He often spoke about his love of Britain, and his desire to own a suit from Saville Row, where, for him, only the best suits, for the highest classes, were made. Mere weeks after his arrival, and not long after finding his first job in London, he managed to do just this, spending a week's wages on a suit that he subsequently wore with pride. That is until, during one evening out with friends, he was subjected to racist taunts and abuse, an experience which left him feeling ashamed, belittled and alone in a country that he then realised was not his home.

Shame is therefore another experience which hampers the identity of the other in these situations. The shame in this case of trying to be the same as, but always being told one will be less than the subject, that they are superior. The student recognised that her father's experience mirrored that of her own during the seminar, so we looked at just how shame had become an aspect of her experience of being the other in a subject's culture. Like the student who felt the need to hide her disability, that sense of otherness, that shame at their difference, plays an important part in unconsciously encouraging the other to comply, to fit in with a cultural, gendered or other narrative of difference which is not their own.

Conversely, for the subject, as Krizan and Johar (2012) saw, shame then becomes the divider between the two sides of narcissism, with envy being a motivator for the need to denigrate the other. Often this sense of envy is so unconscious as to be almost unnoticeable, but much like the competitive students, or the racist chanting of those who put down the student's father over his purchase of a nice suit. Yet, when superiority and envy clash within the psyche, the inability to align the two together can lead some persons, some groups or countries, to want to either dominate or shame the other. Shame therefore becomes an indicator for the subject of its own lack, of that which it desires but does not have, or cannot be. Ultimately, shame becomes the indicator of the subject's own inhumanity over the envied, and therefore objectified, other.

So, for the student in the counselling seminar, who then felt alone and isolated because of her difference, when we explored her echoing of the subject's position, she acknowledged a sense of shame over her difference. A shame which she recognised initially manifested itself in an unconscious anger at her own sense of cultural otherness. This echoes a point Tan (2015) discusses where that shame of one's racialised identity becomes a driver for clients of colour adopting the position of echo. This anger towards oneself often leads clients of colour to avoid persons from their own culture, or like the parents of the client they denigrate those of a similar background, for example criticising others from their home country for not 'fitting in to British culture well enough'. This transgenerational shame of their difference, a shame therefore passed on to the client, meant that for her to raise her difference on her course she had to face this sense of shame. To speak from a more authentic position, to resist the urge to be Narcissus' Echo, the shame of not complying, of being other, she had to find the qualities she needed in order to be more than she felt she could be.

Our unconscious intersectional identity

During one session, the student mentioned that she had to undertake a number of presentations as part of her course, occasionally on her own, but there were also times when she had to work with her colleagues, expressing her distaste for these exercises, as she was always gripped with anxiety. Not long after the student mentioned the approaching assignment, the student presented a dream whereby she was a white woman at the front of the class presenting a topic for the students in the room. Although she knew what she wanted to say, and although she had prepared thoroughly for the seminar, the student still felt a certain sense of imposter syndrome. She complained of not feeling good enough, that she should not be up there, that she was not meant to be a psychotherapist. In the context of this chapter, the importance of this simple dream should not be understated. This client who, even though we were busily exploring her relationship to privilege and otherness, and who was beginning to recognise that her relationship to the subject was an echoing one, also had to sit with the underlying sense of not feeling good enough in relation to her peers.

Although this chapter has explored the conscious, intersectional layering of identity, it should be noted that who we are, the facets of identity that we all carry, are not all held consciously. Such as discussed in psychodynamic psychotherapy, for the child who internalises the good, or bad, parent, the repetition of relational experiences of said mother or father inevitably form a large layer of that child's personality (Mitchell, 1986; Winnicott, 1961). This experience does not end in childhood however and continues throughout life as we reinvent ourselves time and again, learning from, and being mirrored by, those we meet in work, in relationships, in the personal groups and gangs we form and break away from. Even in therapy, one of the aims of the therapist is to be the good enough object which the client, when they are ready, can then internalise and take away, repairing whichever wound brought them into the therapeutic alliance initially.

This is no different when we encounter aspects of otherness, privilege and supremacy. Over time, these too become internalised, meaning that they no longer need to be consciously reactivated externally, and the behaviours inculcated through the experience of being labelled the other, or to holding privilege, are performed without any real knowledge or awareness of their psychological impact upon said master or slave as discussed within the work of Fanon (2005). Understanding internalised experiences of these kinds is nothing new. For example, as discussed in their essays on the internalised impact of sexism Fredrickson and Harrison (2005) considered the negative neurological impact upon women of being objectified. Alternatively, studies have also been conducted which explore the link between internalised racism and increased obesity and high blood pressure (Butler et al., 2002; Tull et al., 1999).

Approaching this though from a more psychotherapeutic perspective, as Lacan (2003) noted, the other is not always external to ourselves. Often, that which we deem to be the shadow, is our own other, that which our egoic sense of self protects us from knowing. This is where the idea of projection became key in my work with the student. As von Franz (1980) recognised when considering projection, just as individuals can project aspects of themselves that they do not like on to persons around them, so too can whole groups do this to other whole groupings, labelling them bad as a means of control over their own, conscious and unconscious, otherness. The unconscious psychological split and casting outwards onto the whiteness of the presenter of that which was deemed 'good' therefore needed to be revealed, recognised and reowned by the student, in order for her to progress.

In our free association exploration of the dream, we looked at just what she thought a white lecturer could do that would have made them appear to be better than her, and what qualities they had that she felt she did not. The student listed such things as confidence, wisdom, the right to be there, power, presence. I reminded the student that, although the dream was playing in to her own fears of being in front of the course, the dream was telling her that she already had the qualities she sought from those she perceived to be in a more authoritative position than herself. The student and I then plotted a path wherein she could begin to acknowledge the varying intersectional layers of her identity whereby she did have authority, where she did have power, knowledge and privilege. Thereby removing her from the position of echo and directing her identity towards one which would ultimately be more authentic, more real and healthier.

References

Andrews, K. (2018). *Back to Black: Retelling Black radicalism for the 21st century*. London: Zed Books.

Appiah, K. A. (2016). Mistaken identities: Creed, country, color, culture. Reith Lectures. London: BBC.

BBC. (2014). Margaret Thatcher's criticism of Brixton riot response revealed. Retrieved from www.bbc.co.uk/news/uk-30600064

Beauvoir, S. de. (2010). *The second sex*. New York: Alfred A. Knopf.

Benjamin, J. (1998). *Shadow of the other*. New York: Routledge.

Bhopal, K. (2018). *White privilege: The myth of a post-racial society*. London: Policy Press.

Biewen, J. (2017). Seeing white (Part 2 How race was made?). Retrieved 20 September 2017, from www.acast.com/cdspodcas/how-race-was-made-seeing-white-part-2

Biewen, J., & Headlee, C. (2018). Men (series 3): Dick move. Retrieved 13 September 2018, from www.sceneonradio.org/episode-47-dick-move-men-part-1/

Bion, W. (1985). Container and contained. *Group Relations Reader, 2*, 127–133.

Brooks, C. (2010). Unidentified allies: Intersections of feminist and transpersonal thought and potential contributions to social change. *International Journal of Transpersonal Studies, 29*(2), 33–57.

Butler, C., Tull, E. S., Chambers, E. C., & Taylor, J. (2002). Internalised racism, body fat distribution, and abnormal fasting glucose among Caribbean women in Dominica, West Indies. *Journal of the National Medical Association, 94*(3), 143–148.

Carastathis, A. (2014). The concept of intersectionality in feminist theory. *Philosophy Compass, 9*(5), 304–314. https://doi.org/10.1111/phc3.12129

Cho, S., Crenshaw, K. W., & Mccall, L. (2013). Toward a field of intersectionality studies: Theory, applications, and praxis. *Signs: Journal of Women in Culture and Society, 38*(4), 785–810.

Collins, P. H., & Bilge, S. (2016). *Intersectionality: Key concepts*. Cambridge: Polity Press.

Cratsley, K. (2015). Revisiting Freud and Kohut on narcissism. *Theory and Psychology, 26*(3), 333–359. https://doi.org/10.1177/0959354316638181

Croxford, R. (2018). Ethnic minority academics earn less than white colleagues. Retrieved on 14 February 2019, from www.bbc.co.uk/news/education-46473269

Di Angelo, R. (2011). White fragility. *International Journal of Critical Pedagogy, 3*(3), 54–70. Retrieved from https://libjournal.uncg.edu/ijcp/article/view/249

Digby, T. O. F. (1992). Political correctness and the fear of feminism. *The Humanist*, March/April, 7–9.

Drazdowski, T. K., Perrin, P. B., Trujillo, M., Sutter, M., Benotsch, E. G., & Snipes, D. J. (2016). Structural equation modeling of the effects of racism, LGBTQ discrimination, and internalized oppression on illicit drug use in LGBTQ people of color. *Drug and Alcool Dependence*. https://doi.org/10.1016/j.drugalcdep.2015.12.029

Duffell, N. (2014). *Wounded leaders: British elitism and the entitlement illusion*. London: Lone Arrow Press.

Fanon, F. (2005). *Black skin, white mask*. (M. Silverman, Ed.). Manchester: Manchester University Press.

Fredrickson, B. L., & Harrison, K. (2005). Throwing like a girl: Self-objectification predicts adolescent girls' motor performance. *Journal of Sport and Social Issues, 29*(1), 79–101. https://doi.org/10.1177/0193723504269878

Gilligan, C. (1982). *In a different voice: Psychological theory and women's development*. Cambridge, MA: Harvard Publishing.

Glen, P. M. J. (2012). Sometimes good guys don't wear white: Morality in the music press, 1967–1983. Thesis submitted for the degree of Doctor of Philosophy, Department of History, University of Sheffield.

Haug, F. (2008). Memory work. *Australian Feminist Studies, 23*(58), 537–541. https://doi.org/10.1080/08164640802433498

HM Government. (2010). *Equality Act 2010,* Chapter 15. Retrieved from https://www.legislation.gov.uk/ukpga/2010/15/pdfs/ukpga_20100015_en.pdf
Homer, S. (2007). *Jacques Lacan: Routledge critical thinkers.* London: Routledge.
Kristeva, J. (1982). *An essay on abjection.* New York: Columbia University Press.
Krizan, Z., & Johar, O. (2012). Envy divides the two faces of narcissism. *Journal of Personality, 80*(5), 1415–1451. https://doi.org/10.1111/j.1467-6494.2012.00767.x
Lacan, J. (2003). *The Cambridge Companion to Lacan.* Ed. J.-M. Rabate. Cambridge: Cambridge University Press. https://doi.org/10.1017/CCOL0521807441
Memmi, A. (1974). *The colonizer and the colonized.* London: Souvenir Press.
Mereish, E. H. (2012). The intersectional invisibility of race and disability status: An exploratory study of health and discrimination facing Asian Americans with disabilities. *Ethnicity and Inequalities in Social Care, 5*(2), 52–60. https://doi.org/10.1108/17570981211286796
Mitchell, J. (1986). *The selected Melanie Klein.* London: Penguin Ltd.
Morrison, A. P. (Ed.). (1986). *Essential papers on narcissism.* New York: New York University Press.
Ovid. (2015). *The Metamorphoses.* Irvine, CA: Xist Publishing.
Said, E. (1993). Representations of an intellectual lecture 2: Holding nations and traditions at bay. Reith Lectures. London: BBC.
Somerville, C. (2015). *Unhealthy attitudes: The treatment of LGBT people within health and social care services.* London: Stonewall. Retrieved from www.stonewall.org.uk/campaign-groups/conversion-therapy
Spivak, G. (1993). Echo. *New Literary History, 24*(1), 17–43.
Tan, T. S. (2015). Race and romance: Understanding students of color in interracial relationships. *The Vermont Connection, 35*(February), 122–129.
Tull, S. E., Wickramasuriya, T., Taylor, J., Smith-Burns, V., Brown, M., Champagnie, G., … & Jordan, O. W. (1999). Relationship of internalized racism to abdominal obesity and blood pressure in Afro-Caribbean women. *Journal of the National Medical Association, 91*(8), 447–452. Retrieved from www.pubmedcentral.nih.gov/articlerender.fcgi?artid=2608441&tool=pmcentrez&rendertype=abstract
Various. (2017). Leading UK psychological professions and Stonewall unite against conversion therapy. Retrieved 19 December 2018, from www.bacp.co.uk/news/2017/16-october-2017-leading-uk-psychological-professions-and-stonewall-unite-against-conversion-therapy/
von Franz, M.-L. (1980). *Projection and Re-collection in Jungian psychology.* London: Open Court Publications.
Weil, A. M., & Piaget, J. (1951). The development in children of the idea of the homeland and of relations to other countries. *International Social Sciences Journal, 3,* 561–578.
Winnicott, D. W. (1961). The theory of the parent–infant relationship. *International Journal of Psycho-Analysis, 1960,* 585–595.

Chapter 13

Embracing the kaleidoscope

Talking about race and racism in clinical psychology

Stephanie Hicks and Catherine Butler

Summary

Race has been defined as 'the notion of a distinct biological type of human being, usually based on skin colour or other physical characteristics' (Delgado et al., 2017, 182). From the early 18th century the essentialist biological notion of race has been used to segregate, exploit and abuse Black and other ethnic minority individuals and establish White power and privilege (Fanon, 1967; Kendi, 2019; Olson, 2005). Prior to the 18th century, concepts of 'race' and racism did not exist in their current form (Kendi, 2019). Although laws now exist against acts such as slavery and racial abuse, White privilege and racism persist to this day (Wood & Patel, 2017). The authors of this chapter are two White, female clinical psychologists. We position ourselves as understanding 'race' to be a social construct that does not exist objectively or biologically in any form, however, we know full well that racism and white supremacy is still prevalent throughout society today, with devastating consequences for those from Black and ethnic minority backgrounds. We therefore use the terms 'race' and 'racism' with this understanding in mind.

Race as a system of power

'Whiteness' is a term used to describe the perceived and enacted superiority of White people in society (Butler et al., 2010). This term refers to race as a system of power and encompasses three aspects: first, White majority group racial identity for those seen by society as fitting with the 'norm'; secondly, racism and bias against those who are not seen as White; and thirdly, racial privilege in which White is the norm against which others are compared (Lyubansky, 2011). Race has been argued to be a 'product of social thought and relations [with] categories that society invents, manipulates, or retires when convenient' (Delgado et al., 2017, 9). Kendi (2019) defines race as 'a power construct of collected or merged difference that lives socially' (p. 35). For example, in cases of violence committed by someone perceived to be White, the act is attributed to the individual; however, if the same act were to be committed by someone perceived to be Black then it can be attributed to some 'characteristics of "them" or "those people"' (Jackson, 2015, 7). This serves to maintain the positive image of being White and the lower status of those seen as Black (Jackson, 2015). The real-world consequences of this system are privilege and advantage for those who fit with the White norm and oppression and abuse towards those who do not (e.g. Delgado et al., 2017; Lyubansky, 2011).

Racism in the UK

Incidents of racism in the day-to-day lives of people from disadvantaged racial groups in the UK are well documented. For example, Black people report that they have to 'work twice as hard to get half as far in life' as they are 'questioned, harassed ... all for essentially "living while black"' (Anderson, 2018, 1). Those from disadvantaged racial groups in the UK are more likely to encounter abuse, be wrongly convicted of shoplifting and be treated differently because of their appearance (Booth & Mohdin, 2018); racism is considered to be 'business as usual' for those oppressed and discriminated against (Benson & Lewis, 2019).

Government figures taken from the Ethnicity Facts and Figures website (www.ethnicity-facts-figures.service.gov.uk) starkly illustrate the real-world inequalities that persist as a result of racism and oppression in the UK. For example: 1) The police stop and search 38 in 1,000 Black people in comparison to only 4 in 1,000 White people, 2) in the NHS Black men are paid 84p for every £1 received by White men, 3) Mixed White and Black Caribbean pupils are three times as likely to be permanently excluded than White British pupils and 4) in 2018 4% of White people were unemployed compared to 7% of people from all other ethnic groups combined (Race Disparity Unit, 2020).

Kendi (2019) argues that racism occurs as a result of racist policy. He describes how this policy embeds the concept that it is specific 'types' of people that are the problem, leading to a vicious cycle of racist ideas: 'Racist ideas make people of colour think less of themselves, which makes them more vulnerable to racist ideas. Racist ideas make White people think more of themselves, which further attracts them to racist ideas' (p. 6). This internalisation of racism is well documented (e.g. Ahmed et al., 2018). For those who identify as Black, this may result in a sense of worthlessness and powerlessness. For those identifying as White this may result in a sense of entitlement and privilege (Bivens, 2005; Fanon, 1967).

Blank et al. (2004) discuss the disconnect in modern society in the way that racism is seemingly frowned upon, and yet racist policy still persists. They describe modern types of racism, such as indirect (e.g. blaming disadvantaged racial groups for their position in society) and ambiguous (e.g. favouring Whites who are in a position of power). Kendi (2019) describes the prevalence of those who pride themselves on rejecting the racist statements of others and yet are in denial of the ways in which they themselves are racist. He argues that 'denial is the heartbeat of racism' (Kendi, 2019, 9), as those who describe themselves as 'not racist' are allowing racial inequalities to persist through inaction; he asserts that one can only be racist or 'anti-racist' (i.e., actively fighting racism).

The terms 'post-racial' and 'colour-blind' have been used to describe a society that is free from racial inequality, however these ideas have been strongly refuted (e.g. Hirsch, 2018; Ikuenobe, 2013; Kendi, 2019; Prajapati et al., 2019). Colour-blind refers to a virtue in which skin colour is viewed as irrelevant in relation to the worth of a person (Jones, 2016). Post-racial refers to a society that no longer needs to discuss race, as racism no longer exists (Ikuenobe, 2013). It has been argued that these terms only perpetuate the myth of racial equality, resulting in denial and inaction in response to persistent racist policy and abuse (Hirsch, 2018; Kendi, 2019; The Runnymede Trust, 2016). Instead, the literature describes the undeniable prevalence of racism and the way in which society continues to be structured around race (e.g. Ikuenobe, 2013).

Race and mental health

It is well-established that higher rates of distress exist in disadvantaged racial groups as a result of persistent racism (e.g. Department of Health, 2005; Kutchins & Kirk, 1999; Memon et al., 2016; Pascoe & Smart Richman, 2009). Historically, psychiatric diagnoses have been used by psychologists and psychiatrists to justify oppression and reinforce the superiority of White people by wrongly attributing 'disorders' to individuals as a result of their perceived race (Fanon, 1967). For example, the prevalence of certain diagnoses (such as psychosis) is recorded as abnormally high in disadvantaged racial groups and identical behaviours or experiences are observed as more severe when seen in African Americans compared to those who are White (Kutchins & Kirk, 1999).

For those seeking support, there are race-related barriers in accessing both mental health services and the psychological therapies offered. Recent research shows how individuals from disadvantaged racial groups face multiple barriers in accessing services as they experience insensitivity, racist abuse and a power imbalance between themselves and White clinicians (Memon et al., 2016). These barriers have persisted for many years despite government efforts to tackle this, for example with the 'Delivering Race Equality in Mental Health Care' action plan (Department of Health, 2005).

In relation to treatment, the behaviour of clinicians towards patients is informed by the racial category which they perceive the patient as 'belonging to'. Campbell (2012) describes how attributing a racial group to others is a way for White clinicians to ensure our survival in a world based on racist power. He describes an ingrained desire to form relationships which continue to enhance our own position in some way, and by default this results in a position of powerlessness for the 'other'. For example, a White clinical psychologist is likely to perpetuate patterns of racial power and White privilege in the therapy room when working with individuals from disadvantaged racial groups. The client may not feel that the therapeutic space is safe or respectful as a result, leading to emotions such as anger and distress (Pascoe & Smart Richman, 2009).

This is only a brief introduction to the complex interaction between race and mental health; however it illustrates the importance of clinical psychologists understanding race and its impact on our work. It would be a travesty not to include race in our formulations and therapeutic work with clients, and therefore we need to be able to talk about race and acknowledge the ways in which we perpetuate racist power.

Racism in clinical psychology

Despite its importance, clinical psychologists are rarely trained in addressing and working directly with race as the profession is embedded in Whiteness (Wood & Patel, 2019). There is a lack of racial diversity within the profession and we are blinded by a Eurocentric and US-centred evidence base. The majority of theories are written by White academics and practitioners and the 'evidence' which backs up these theories is based on studies of White people (Adetimole et al., 2005; Patel, 2003; Patel & Fatimilehin, 2005; Turpin & Coleman, 2010; Wood & Patel, 2017).

On clinical psychology training courses, those with a minority racial status are still seen as 'other', with an assumption of inferiority in difference (Adetimole et al., 2005). For the few trainees who identify as Black, the profession is viewed as one which continues to reinforce inequalities and does not represent the communities it attempts to serve (Olubunmi & Odusanya, 2016). This may be a legacy of the way in which the institution of therapy has maintained racist structures, with mental health diagnoses being used to discriminate against and oppress those from minority racial groups (Fernando, 2017). Through collective Whiteness, clinical psychologists are likely to have 'the privilege to live … without ever needing to be aware of [their] whiteness and how it might be impacting their life' (Lyubansky, 2011), or indeed on the lives of others.

It may feel uncomfortable for White clinical psychologists to start discussions about race, yet without meaningful action racism will persist in clinical psychology (Wood & Patel, 2019). Efforts are already being made to address issues of race and racism in clinical psychology (e.g. Berg et al., 2019), however these efforts are not widespread. Establishing a framework within which clinical psychologists can begin to understand and talk about race may be a step towards more widespread change.

Racial inconsistency

For many years social institutions have asked individuals to select a racial identity from a list of categories (Rockquemore & Brunsma, 2002). This enables these institutions to process race (e.g., collect data on protected characteristics), but it could be argued that this ensures the continuation of an oppressive colonial society as race is viewed as a static characteristic (Blank et al., 2004; Fanon, 1967). With the rise of multicultural communities in the UK, society's categories no longer seem to fit for a growing number of people. Whilst acknowledging the profound impact of race, researchers in fields such as sociology are questioning how race should be understood in relation to the categories used (e.g. Boonzaier & van Niekerk, 2019; Delgado et al., 2017; Fanon, 1967; Jackson, 2009; Roth, 2016).

Roth (2016) suggests these categories are descriptive of multiple dimensions of race, with individuals potentially being classified or self-identifying differently within each dimension. For example:

> Salvador, a restaurant worker in New York, identifies his race as Puerto Rican. Phenotypically, he is dark-skinned with indigenous features, leading some Americans to view him as Black. He believes that Americans view him as Hispanic, based on his accent and name. Yet on the census, Salvador checks White for his race because no listed options fits his identity and in Puerto Rico his mixed racial ancestry allowed him to consider himself closer to White than to Black.
>
> (Roth, 2016, pp. 1310–1311)

Roth (2016) describes how an individual's race may be considered as their racial identity, racial self-classification, observed race, reflected race, phenotype and racial ancestry. This is supported by studies which suggest 'race is changeable, contextual and multi-dimensional' (Boda, 2018, 29), whilst acknowledging the impact and existence of racism and oppression (Delgado et al., 2017).

Roth (2016) describes race within these dimensions as fluid across both time and context, highlighting that race is not static but 'inconsistent'. Her term 'racial inconsistency' will be used throughout this chapter to explore race as a fluid and multi-dimensional construct.

The concept of racial inconsistency has similarities to intersectionality (Crenshaw, 1989) – a model commonly used in law, sociology, race studies, feminism and increasingly used in clinical psychology to understand the impact of overlapping individual characteristics (e.g., gender). For example, both racial inconsistency and intersectionality refer to individual characteristics being fluid and changeable in their impact depending on their interaction with other aspects of that individual's identity and the societal structures and policies the individual comes up against. Acknowledging that scaffolding can support learning (Vygotsky, 1978), it is possible that racial inconsistency may be a useful framework for clinical psychologists to begin to understand and talk about race, as there are theoretical similarities to a model already used in the profession.

Purpose of this chapter

As professionals working in the UK context of providing a healthcare system for all (Department of Health, 2005; Wood & Patel, 2017), this chapter aims to support clinical psychologists to understand and work with race and racism. Using a systematic review, the authors hope to explore whether racial inconsistency may be a useful framework for clinical psychologists to start conversations on this topic and then begin to address embedded racism in the profession.

Systematic literature review

A systematic search of the literature was conducted using IBSS, APA Psycnet, Embase and Web of Science using the search terms 'race OR racial' AND 'fluid OR fluidity OR dimension OR dimensions' AND 'identit* OR experience*'. The initial 712 papers were screened by title (616 excluded), abstract (75 excluded) and full text (15 excluded) using four exclusion criteria: 1) Literature using a quantitative methodology or approach, 2) written in a language other than English, 3) literature that considers race as an essential characteristic of the individual, 4) literature that does not conceptualise race as a fluid or multi-dimensional construct. The reference lists of the remaining seven papers were then searched by hand for any further relevant papers, resulting in a total of 12 papers for review. A quality assessment of the papers was completed using the Critical Appraisal Skills Programme (CASP) qualitative checklist (CASP, 2017) and all articles were then included as they were all seen to have value for the synthesis.

The 12 papers included in the synthesis are summarised below.

- Brubaker (2016) offers a theoretical discussion exploring the concepts of 'transgender' and 'transracial', arguing that thinking within a 'trans' framework can support discussion and understanding around the construct of race. There is a suggestion that society is moving towards a more fluid definition of racial identity.
- Campbell and others (2016) present an editorial piece introducing a special issue of the journal on the measurement and analysis of varying components of race. They summarise the articles and consider wider implications in terms of research and social inequality. .
- Frable (1997) reviews theoretical psychological literature on gender, racial, ethnic, sexual and class identities. The paper discusses how these are fluid and multi-dimensional but generally considered in isolation in research.
- Jackson (2009) uses a narrative approach to explore identity formation in ten multiracial adults with a rigorous line-by-line transcript analysis. The categories of 1) racism and discrimination, 2) social influence and 3) environmental context are described and discussed.
- In 2012 Jackson used the narrative approach to explore the identity experiences of ten multiracial adults. Paradigmatic analysis of narratives used themes of 1) shifting racial/ethnic expressions, 2) racial/ethnic ambiguity, 3) feeling like an outsider, 4) seeking community and 5) racial resistance.

- Morning (2018) offers an opinion piece which brings together recent episodes of public debate on racial identity. The article argues for four new types of race membership – genetic, cosmetic, emotive and constructed.
- Rocha (2018) contrasts the experiences of racial classification for 40 individuals of mixed racial identities in New Zealand and Singapore and discusses their experiences of navigating strict and fluid forms of classification.
- Roth's (2016) theoretical paper discusses literature on the multiple dimensions of race. A novel theoretical model is presented for understanding racial fluidity and inconsistency. The implications of this are discussed in relation to research.
- Snipp's (1997) discussion piece explores race moving from a fixed to an ambiguous construct and considers problems this creates in American society. The discussion is set in the context of Native Americans.
- Song and Hashem (2010) interview 16 East Asian/White individuals around whether 'best single-race' survey questions reflect their feelings of belonging to a racial group. They offer a summary of responses with conclusions made in relation to interpretation of the responses.
- Wilson's (1984) theoretical paper looks at issues relating to the categorisation of 'mixed race' children in Britain and explores theories around the definition of 'mixed race', racial structure in Britain and situational ethnicity.
- Finally, Okamura (1981) offers a review and synthesis of theories from social anthropologists around the relevance of situational factors in the analysis of ethnicity.

Analysis and synthesis

A meta-ethnographic method (Noblit & Hare, 1988) was used, following the method described by Malpass et al. (2009). This method was chosen to gain both breadth and depth of understanding around this complex subject (Siddaway et al., 2019). In summary, the papers were read and reread chronologically, with notes and a conceptual map made on any second-order constructs (an interpretation of what is discussed in each paper). The second-order constructs across all papers were then collated into a table to feed into the development of third-order constructs (an interpretation of the intentions of the original authors). This table grouped and framed the second-order constructs as necessary to account for the interpretation of each construct across all the papers in which it appeared. A lines-of-argument synthesis was then used to develop the third-order constructs. This type of synthesis is described by Noblit and Hare (1988) as a way of inferring 'what we can say about the whole, based on the selective studies of its parts' (p. 63).

Three third-order constructs were established from the original papers: 1) dimensionality of race, 2) racial structure of society and 3) racial identity and the individual.

Dimensionality

Race was consistently described as a social construct – something we 'do' as a society rather than something that individuals 'are'. The papers describe how race is not unitary or fixed, but multi-dimensional. Race is seen as having a wealth of possible dimensions, including (but not limited to): self-assigned racial identity, the race ascribed by others based on appearance, genetic racial ancestry or racial classification on legal documentation. With regards to racial inconsistency, the possibility of an individual being classified differently across different dimensions of race was identified.

The papers discuss how these dimensions of race do not exist exclusively, but intersect and interact with one another. In this way, these papers view race as fluid – changeable across time and situations depending on a range of contextual factors. Individuals are therefore able to hold multiple racial identities simultaneously or potentially hold a more ambiguous racial identity that may not align with any defined category.

The racial structure of society

Racial classification is described as an organising principle of society, as we look to understand other people. Inequality in power is seen as a key factor in the development of racial identity as it establishes a strong sense of 'us and them'. The papers describe how racial classification is used as a method of societal control, marginalising disadvantaged racial groups and increasing White power and privilege.

Race may not always be the most salient and relevant factor guiding interactions in society. The papers suggest that other aspects of identity (e.g. class, gender, sexuality) may at times be seen as more relevant in determining a sense of 'us and them', however these aspects of identity will always intersect. The relationship between both racial and other aspects of identity is therefore complex in how they may interact and intersect to define an individual's sense of self within society, their behaviour within it and how society responds to them.

Several papers describe how the concept of race has changed in recent years, from one based on fixed and stable heredity to one of more ambiguous kinship and belonging (for example, in the case of Rachel Dolezal; Brubaker, 2016). As this change progresses, racial categories used historically in research and public policy are becoming more complex and nuanced. This is potentially problematic as there is less clarity in the concept of a racial minority, making it difficult to draw evidence-based conclusions from research on inequality and allocate scarce resources to address oppression.

The papers described oppression and racist abuse as a common experience for individuals who are perceived by society as a racial minority. These negative experiences have an impact on psychological well-being, for example, individuals not being understood and being disconnected from others.

The papers also describe how racially disadvantaged individuals are likely to seek safety and a sense of community with other people who share similar oppressive experiences in relation to race. In particular, this may occur for individuals who are labelled by society as a race which they do not identify with.

Alternatively, individuals may want to seek safety as they hold a racial identity that is subject to criticism and policing in society/media (e.g. Rachel Dolezal being trans-racial; Brubaker, 2016). The papers also discussed a post-racial stance of 'racial resistance' being held by some groups, in which they actively reject any form of racial classification or categorisation being used to label them as belonging to a certain racial group.

Racial identity and the individual

These papers describe how we look for racial sameness and difference in order to understand the social world around us. In classifying and seeking out others who we perceive to be like 'us', and distancing ourselves from those who we see as different ('them'), we are able to build our own racial identity and develop relationships with those who share similar racial experiences. This may also result in a sense of 'belonging' to a certain racial category and the internalisation of characteristics associated with that category (e.g. power or powerlessness).

The papers describe how the racial classification of the self and others can have an effect on both the behaviour and well-being of individuals. With classification of the self and others comes a deeper understanding of where power lies in relation to race. This understanding influences behaviour in social situations, which may then reflect existing racial inequality (e.g. in the case of internalised racism). Well-being is also affected in relation to the racial experiences of individuals. The papers tended to focus on negative experiences (e.g. oppression) of those who are seen as Black; although it was acknowledged that racial experiences could have both a positive and negative impact.

The papers explored how the fluidity and multi-dimensionality of race may compound the effect of negative racial experiences. As race may change across dimensions, over time and context, these experiences may be directed towards multiple dimensions of a person's racial identity or exist in some contexts but not others.

In the past, race has been understood as a fixed construct and racial classification was seen by some as a true reflection of racial identity. These papers present an alternative view, describing racial identity as developing within a historical, societal and environmental context. The papers discuss a range of both structural and cognitive influences on individual racial identity development.

Structural influences could include stories of racial identity from family or friends, historical narratives from wider society or current experiences of oppression and racist discrimination at the hands of racist policy. Cognitive influences may include our interpretation of the behaviour of others, beliefs about race or comparisons of our self with others.

An examination of racial inconsistency

By completing this review the authors hoped to explore racial inconsistency as a framework within which clinical psychologists can begin to understand and talk about race and racism. It is hoped that by discussing racial inconsistency in the context of an existing model (e.g. intersectionality; Crenshaw, 1989), conversations within clinical psychology may also be scaffolded in a way that brings about more widespread change.

Racial inconsistency and intersectionality

Intersectionality (Crenshaw, 1989) is a critical race feminist theory based on the following premises: 1) that people live multiple layered identities, 2) that this combination of identities results in a unique combination of discrimination, disadvantage, power and privilege, and 3) that the experiences associated with these identities are not a additive, but distinctly different in their impact on the individual (Collins, 2000). This model was chosen as it challenges categorical models of thinking and is commonly used by clinical psychologists to work with discrimination by informing our discussions with clients and the development of formulations (e.g. Brah & Pheonix, 2004; Diamond & Butterworth, 2008).

Within the framework of racial inconsistency, race can be understood as a multi-dimensional social construct with inconsistent dimensions which intersect and interact in a way that is fluid and changeable. Each dimension of race could be understood as combining and interacting to oppress or privilege individuals in unique and multiple ways (Butler, 2015). The multiple dimensions of race alone could therefore be understood as intersectional, alongside the intersection of these dimensions with other areas of identity (e.g. gender, class, sexual orientation).

Racial inconsistency should be understood in the context of a society which is structured by race. Racial hierarchy perpetuates White privilege in society, with oppression and racist abuse being a regular occurrence for individuals from disadvantaged racial groups. Racial inequality is understood as being a key factor in the development of racial identity and racial classification is used as a means of societal control. Depending on each individual's unique experience, the way in which racism is experienced will differ, for example, black men may experience more physical brutality through racism than black women (Ahmed et al., 2018). As a result, those from disadvantaged racial groups may choose to seek safety with those who have similar experiences or take on a post-racial perspective and reject race completely.

We seek out others who share similar experiences of race and can develop a strong sense of belonging to a racial category. Racial inconsistency may compound negative experiences of race or alternatively act as a protective factor against psychological distress. A range of cognitive and structural factors may contribute to the development of racial identity; creating a very complex picture when trying to understand this with individual clients. In any social interaction, multiple dimensions of racial identity could be understood as intersecting across multiple individuals to create a totally unique racial experience for those involved. Each social interaction would then be a kaleidoscope of complex and unique experiences in relation to race as these dimensions shift and change.

Society is not post racial or colour-blind but continues to be structured by race. This structure plays a role in the development of racial identity, but also results in the racist actions and ideas which perpetuate racist abuse for those from disadvantaged racial groups. Claims to a post-racial society have emerged at a time in which society is moving away from the idea of race as a fixed and stable construct (e.g. racial inconsistency), yet 'post-racial strategy makes no sense in our racist world' (Kendi, 2019, 54).

> But for all of that life-shaping power, race is a mirage, which doesn't lessen its force. We are what we see ourselves as, whether what we see exists or not. We are what people see us as, whether what they see exists or not. What people see in themselves and others has meaning and manifests itself in ideas and actions and policies, even if what they are seeing is an illusion.
>
> (Kendi, 2019, 37)

This quote describes the way in which race can be considered *both* as a powerful and influential force in our lives *and* as an inconsistent, intersectional and dynamic social construct. Racial inconsistency may therefore be a useful way in which to understand this mirage so long as it is not aligned with the idea that society is 'post-racial' or 'colour-blind'. In line with intersectionality, race can be understood as inconsistent whilst acknowledging the existence and impact of racism and oppression.

Embracing the kaleidoscope

Racial inconsistency may be a useful framework for clinical psychologists to talk about race and racism in relation to individual well-being, wider society, public policy and research. Racial inconsistency accounts for a wide range of ways in which race may impact on psychological well-being and can be understood within the existing theoretical framework of intersectionality.

The multiple dimensions of race could provide many footholds for perpetuating social inequality and create a complex picture in trying to understand individual experiences of oppression, how that oppression is maintained and the psychological impact it has on the individual, as well as ways that clinical psychologists might directly challenge such oppression.

Racial inconsistency presents race as a complex social construct with real-world consequences and exists as a viable concept set apart from the myth of a post-racial or colour-blind society. It is hoped that, with a framework with which to understand race, clinical psychologists may feel more confident to start conversations with both clients and colleagues on this topic, as well as find ways to make tangible difference in the lives of individuals and communities.

In starting these conversations it is important to embrace the kaleidoscope of racial inconsistency and take a step away from 'knowing' (Sarantakis, 2017). This is in contrast to the various papers written about 'achieving' cultural competencies (e.g. Geerlings et al., 2018), which imply that race is something which can be fully understood. A stance of cultural humility (Tervalon & Murray-Garcia, 1998) is suggested, in which White clinicians are open to the values of others rather than being held to the superiority of their own: 'just don't forget that you can never know what it is like to be black' (Campbell, 2012, 40).

It will also be important for clinical psychologists to step out of isolation in potentially safe communities of people like 'us' and step out into conversations about race with all stakeholders in order to challenge the current consensus (Berg et al., 2019; Kagan et al., 2011). It is hoped by the authors that as clinical psychologists build up competence in talking about race, they may begin to take stronger anti-racist actions against racism and oppression (Kendi, 2019).

Reynolds (2011) describes how those in the helping professions are well-placed for justice-doing, meaning that we can 'work to change the real conditions of people's lives rather than helping them to adjust to oppression' (p. 29); however clinical psychologists specifically will be used to working within a system which discriminates against minority racial groups (Fernando, 2017). There may be a fine line between trying to work in solidarity as an ally with disadvantaged racial groups (Droogendyk et al., 2016; Reynolds, 2013) and being blind to the 'oppressive potential of well-meant performances of care' (Parker, 2019, 7). It is possible that at times the most effective action will be to simply to listen from a position of humility, allowing for a change in power relations so that racially disadvantaged individuals can step forward with their own knowledge and expertise (Parker, 2019).

We acknowledge that the suggestions presented here are only a selection of ideas from authors who consistently identify as White clinical psychologists across time and place. Despite the best efforts to include comments and considerations of those who are experts by either experience or profession, this chapter cannot claim to reflect the diverse views of those with experiences of race different to our own. We also acknowledge that as White clinical psychologists there are many times when we continue to engage with racist policy, use racist language or reinforce racism. We assume this chapter will be no exception despite our intention to encourage our profession to talk about race and racism and take on an anti-racist stance (Kendi, 2019). All we hope is that by stepping out into conversations about race we may be able to inspire other clinical psychologists in the UK to do the same, as well as to continue to develop ourselves.

Racial inconsistency as a framework

Racial inconsistency is a useful framework within which clinical psychologists can continue to understand and talk about race, hopefully going on to inspire anti-racist action from the position of power and privilege that we hold. Through the kaleidoscopic lens of racial inconsistency, race can be understood as fluid and multi-dimensional, resulting in complex and dynamic experiences for individuals. These experiences can be understood as relating to systems of power and White supremacy that impact the well-being of individuals. Provided that racial inconsistency is not utilised as part of a post-racial or colour-blind perspective, it could support more clinical psychologists in an understanding of the complexities of race and racism while acting as allies against oppressive practice and discrimination.

Clinical psychologists should also consider the way in which our profession has developed from a place of White power and privilege. More clinical psychologists need to decolonise their therapeutic practice, research and training by changing practice to address and attend to race. By doing this we may be able to improve the relevance of clinical psychology for the multicultural UK population, effectively support individuals with a variety of racial experiences and engage in more dialogical conversation and anti-racist action in the community.

References

Adetimole, F., Afuape, T., & Vara, R. (2005). The impact of racism on the experience of training on a clinical psychology course: Reflections from three Black trainees. *Clinical Psychology Forum, 48*, 11–15.

Ahmed, K., Aziz, S., Batchelor-Hunt, N., Shaheen, F., & Harker, J. (2018). Racial bias in Britain – what it feels like. *The Guardian* (online). Retrieved 28 August 2019.

Anderson, E. (2018). This is what it feels like to be black in white spaces. *The Guardian* (online). Retrieved 28 August 2019.

Benson, M., & Lewis, C. (2019). Brexit, British people of colour in the EU-27 and everyday racism in Britain and Europe. *Ethnic and Racial Studies, 42*(13), 2211–2228.

Berg, K., Romero, M. C., Harper, D., Patel, N., Patel, T., Rees, N., & Smith, R. (2019). Why are we still talking about race. *Clinical Psychology Forum, 323*, 8–13.

Bivens, D. K. (2005). What is internalised racism? In M. Potapchuk, S. Leiderman, D. Bivens, & B. Major (Eds.). *Flipping the script: White priviledge and community building* (pp. 43–51). Silver Spring, MD: MP Associates.

Blank, R. M., Dabady, M., & Citro, C. F. (2004). Theories of discrimination. In R. M. Blank, M. Dabady & C. F. Citro (Eds.). *Measuring racial discrimination*. Washington, DC: National Academies Press.

Boda, Z. (2018). Social influence on observed race. *Sociological Science, 5*, 29–57.

Boonzaier, F., & van Niekerk, T. (2019). Introducing decolonial feminist community psychology. In F. Boonzaier & T. van Niekerk (Eds.). *Decolonial feminist community psychology* (pp. 1–10). Cham: Springer.

Booth, R., & Mohdin, A. (2018). Revealed: The stark evidence of everyday racial bias in Britain. *The Guardian* (online). Retrieved 28 August 2019.

Brah, A., & Pheonix, A. (2004). Ain't I a woman? Revisiting intersectionality. *Journal of International Women's Studies, 5*(3), 75–86.

Brubaker, R. (2016). *Trans: Gender and race in an age of unsettled identities*. Princeton, NJ: Princeton University Press.

Butler, C. (2015). Intersectionality in family therapy training: Inviting students to embrace the complexities of lived experience. *Journal of Family Therapy, 37*, 583–589.

Butler, C., das Nair, R., & Thomas, S. (2010). The colour of queer. In L. Moon (Ed.). *Counselling ideologies: Queer challenges to heteronormativity*. Farnham: Ashgate.

Campbell, D. (2012). Can we tolerate the relationships that race compels? In I. B. Krause (Ed.). *Culture and reflexivity in systemic psychotherapy: Mutual perspectives* (pp. 52–65). London: Karnac Books Ltd.

Campbell, M. E., Bratter, J. L., & Roth, W. D. (2016). Measuring the diverging components of race: An introduction. *American Behavioral Scientist, 60*(4), 381–389.

Collins, P. H. (2000). *Black feminist thought: Knowledge, consciousness, and the politics of empowerment (perspectives on gender)*. New York: Routledge.

Crenshaw, K. (1989). Demarginalizing the intersection of race and sex: A black feminist critique of antidiscrimination doctrine, feminist theory, and anti-racist politics. *University of Chicago Legal Forum, 140*, 139–167.

Critical Appraisal Skills Programme. (2017). CASP qualititative checklist. Retrieved from https://casp-uk.net/casp-tools-checklists/

Delgado, R., Jean, S., & Harris, A. (2017). *Critical race theory: An introduction* (3rd ed.). New York: New York University Press.

Department of Health. (2005). *Delivering race equality in mental health care: An action plan for reform inside and outside services and the government's response to the independent inquiry into the death of David Bennett*. London: Department of Health.

Diamond, L. M., & Butterworth, M. (2008). Questioning gender and sexual identity: Dynamic links over time. *Sex Roles, 59*, 365–376.

Droogendyk, L., Wright, S. C., Lubensky, M., & Louis, W. R. (2016). Acting in solidarity: Cross-group contact between disadvantaged group members and advantaged group allies. *Journal of Social Issues, 72*(2), 315–334.

Fanon, F. (1967). *Black skin, white masks*. New York: Grove Press.

Fernando, S. (2017). *Institutional racism in psychiatry and clinical psychology*. London: Palgrave Macmillan.

Frable, D. E. S. (1997). Gender, racial, ethnic, sexual, and class identities. *Annual Review of Psychology, 48*, 139–162.

Geerlings, L. R. C., Thompson, C. L., Bouma, R., & Hawkins, R. (2018). Cultural competence in clinical psychology training: A qualitative investigation of student and academic experiences. *Australian Psychologist, 53*(2), 161–170.

Hirsch, A. M. (2018). I've had enough of white people who try to deny my experience. *The Guardian* (online). Retrieved 28 August 2019.

Ikuenobe, P. (2013). Conceptualizing and theorizing about the idea of a 'post-racial' era. *Journal for the Theory of Social Behaviour, 43*(4), 446–468.

Jackson, K. F. (2009). Beyond race: Examining the facets of multiracial identity through a life-span developmental lens. *Journal of Ethnic and Cultural Diversity in Social Work, 18*(4), 293–310.

Jackson, K. F. (2012). Living the multiracial experience: Shifting racial expressions, resisting race and seeking community. *Qualitative Social Work, 11*(1), 42–60.

Jackson, S. A. (2015). Theorising race, class and gender studies. In S. A. Jackson (Ed.). *Routledge international handbook of race, class and gender* (pp. 1–30). New York: Routledge.

Jones, J. M. (2016). The colour-blind racial approach: Does race really matter? In H. A. Neville, M. E. Gallardo, & D. W. Sue (Eds.). *The myth of racial colour blindness: Manifestations, dynamics, and impact* (pp. 39–52). Washington, DC: American Psychological Association.

Kagan, C., Burton, M., Duckett, P., Lawthom, R., & Siddiquee, A. (2011). *Critical community psychology*. Oxford: British Psychological Society and Blackwell Publishing Ltd.

Kendi, I. X. (2019). *How to be an anti-racist*. London: Penguin Random House.

Kutchins, H., & Kirk, S. A. (1999). The enduring legacy of racisim in the diagnosis of mental disorders. In H. Kutchins & S. A. Kirk (Eds.). *Making us crazy: DSM – the psychiatric bible and the creation of mental disorders*. New York: Free Press.

Lyubansky, M. (2011). The meaning of Whiteness. Retrieved 22 July 2019, from www.psychologytoday.com/gb/blog/between-the-lines/201112/the-meaning-whiteness

Malpass, A., Shaw, A., Sharp, D., Walter, F., Feder, G., Ridd, M., & Kessler, D. (2009). 'Medication career' or 'moral career'? The two sides of managing antidepressants: A meta-ethnography of patients' experience of antidepressants. *Social Science and Medicine, 68*(1), 154–168.

Memon, A., Taylor, K., Mohebati, L. M., Sundin, J., Cooper, M., Scanlon, T., & de Visser, R. (2016). Perceived barriers to accessing mental health services among black and minority ethnic (BME) communities: A qualitative study in Southeast England. *British Medical Journal Open, 6*(11), e012337.

Morning, A. (2018). Kaleidoscope: Contested identities and new forms of race membership. *Ethnic and Racial Studies, 41*(6), 1055–1073.

Noblit, G. W., & Hare, R. D. (1988). *Meta-ethnography: Synthesizing qualitative studies* (vol. 11). Thousand Oaks, CA: Sage.

Okamura, J. (1981). Situational ethnicity. *Ethnic and Racial Studies, 4*(4), 452–465.

Olson, J. (2005). W. E. B. Du Bois and the race concept. *Souls,* 7(3–4), 118–128.

Olubunmi, S., & Odusanya, E. (2016). The experience of qualified BME clinical psychologists: An interpretative phenomenological and repertory grid analysis. Doctorate of Clinical Psychology, University of Hertfordshire.

Parker, J. (2019). Towards systemic praxis for social change: The politics of practice and practices of hope. *Context, 164*, 6–9.

Pascoe, E. A., & Smart Richman, L. (2009). Perceived discrimination and health: A meta-analytic review. *Psychological Bulletin, 135*(4), 531–554.

Patel, N. (2003). Clinical psychology: Reinforcing inequalities or facilitating empowerment? *International Journal of Human Rights,* 7(1), 16–39.

Patel, N., & Fatimilehin, I. (2005). Racism and clinical psychology: What's changed? *Clinical Psychology Forum, 48*, 20–23.

Prajapati, R., Kadir, S., & King, S. (2019). Dealing with racism within clinical psychology training: Reflections of BAME trainee clinical psychologists. *Clinical Psychology Forum, 323*, 20–24.

Race Disparity Unit (2020). Ethnicity facts and figures. Retrieved 8 July 2020 from www.ethnicity-facts-figures.service.gov.uk

Reynolds, V. (2011). Resisting burnout with justice doing. *International Journal of Narrative Therapy and Community Work, 4*, 27–45.

Reynolds, V. (2013). 'Leaning in' as imperfect allies in community work. *Narrative and Conflict: Explorations of Theory and Practice, 1*(1), 53–75.

Rocha, Z. L. (2018). Strict versus flexible categorizations of mixedness: Classifying mixed race in Singapore and New Zealand. *Social Identities, 25*(3), 310–326.

Rockquemore, K. A., & Brunsma, D. L. (2002). Socially embedded identities: Theories, typologies, and processes of racial identity among black/white biracials. *Sociological Quarterly, 43*(3), 335–356.

Roth, W. D. (2016). The multiple dimensions of race. *Ethnic and Racial Studies, 39*(8), 1310–1338.

The Runnymede Trust. (2016). *UK NGOs' alternative report: Submission to the UN Committee on the Elimination of Racial Discrimination with regard to the UK Government's 21st to 23rd periodic reports*. London: The Runnymede Trust.

Sarantakis, N. P. (2017). Reflections on an anti-discriminatory stance in psychotherapy. *Journal of Contemporary Psychotherapy, 47*(2), 135–140.

Siddaway, A. P., Wood, A. M., & Hedges, L. V. (2019). How to do a systematic review: A best practice guide for conducting and reporting narrative reviews, meta-analyses, and meta-syntheses. *Annual Review of Psychology, 70*, 747–770.

Snipp, C. M. (1997). Some observations about racial boundaries and the experiences of American Indians. *Ethnic and Racial Studies, 20*(4), 667–689.

Song, M., & Hashem, F. (2010). What does "White" mean? Interpreting the choice of "race" by mixed race young people in Britain. *Sociological Perspectives, 53*(2), 287–292.

Tervalon, M., & Murray-Garcia, J. (1998). Cultural humility versus cultural competence: A critical distinction in defining physician training outcomes in multicultural education. *Journal of Health Care for the Poor and Underserved, 9*(2), 117–125.

Turpin, G., & Coleman, G. (2010). Clinical psychology and diversity: Progress and continuing challenges. *Psychology Learning and Teaching, 9*(2), 17–27.

Vygotsky, L. S. (1978). *Mind in society: The development of higher psychological processes*. Cambridge, MA: Harvard University Press.

Wilson, A. (1984). 'Mixed race' children in British society: Some theoretical considerations. *British Journal of Sociology, 35*(1), 42–61.

Wood, N., & Patel, N. (2017). On addressing 'whiteness' during clinical psychology training. *South African Journal of Psychology, 47*(3), 280–291.

Wood, N., & Patel, N. (2019). Special issue: Racism during training in clinical psychology. *Clinical Psychology Forum, 323*, 1–52.

Name index

Abraham, K. 103
Adler, A. 102
Asch 103
Avaristo, B. 154, 158

Bandler, R. 103
Beck, A. 103, 105
Berke, J. 104, 108
Berne, E. 103, 105
Bettleheim, B. 102
Bleasdale, Alan 64
Boring, E.G. 22–3
Bowie, David 168
Breuer, J. 102

Campbell, Bronwyn 114, 116
Cartwright, S. 72–4, 81–2
Chamberlin, Judi 70, 82
Chesterton, G.K. 58, 67
Connolly, V. 6
Crenshaw, K. 88, 96, 165, 174, 180, 185, 189
Cruikshank, G. 66

Davis, Eliza 59
Di Angelo, R. 170, 174
Dickens, C. 57–68
Dudgeon, P. 46, 48, 49, 55, 94, 97, 141, 143

Eisner, W. 65–7
Eitingon, M. 103
Ellis, A. 103
Erikson, E. 102

Fagin 58–61, 64–8
Fanon, F. 173, 174, 175, 177, 179
Ferenczi, S. 103
Fernando, S. 16, 25, 27, 132, 143, 179, 187, 189
Festinger, L. 103
Foucault, M. 52, 55, 58, 88, 97, 102
Frankl, V. 103, 108
Freire, P. 141, 144
Frenkel-Brunswik, E. 103
Freud, A. 102
Freud, S. 101, 109, 162
Fromm, E. 104

Galton, F. 5, 88
Geertz, C. 3, 14, 151, 158
Guinness, Alec 58

Harwood, Ronald 65
Heinroth, J.C.A. 105, 109
Henry III 63
Hillel (c. 110 BCE – 10 CE) 108
Hitler, A. 17, 106–7

Janov, A. 103
Jastrow, J. 103
Jones, E. 103, 108
Jones, T. 154, 158
Jung, C.G. 103, 162

Kant, Emmanuel. 105
Kendi, I.X. 176–188, 190
Kingsley, Sir Ben. 64, 67
Klein, M. 102
Kohlberg, L. 103

Lacan, J. 162, 167, 170, 173, 175
Laing, R. 104
Lawrence, Stephen. 27, 40
Lean, David. 60
Lewin, K. 103

Lifton, R. J. 104, 107, 109
Little St Hugh of Lincoln 61–3, 68

Maslow, A. 103
Marx, K. 107, 118, 129
Moodley, R. 132–3, 141, 145

Nancy 60–1

Ovid (43 BCE – 17/18 CE) 163, 175

Paris, Matthew. 62
Patel, N. 9, 15, 32, 41, 147, 158, 179, 188, 190, 191
Perls, F. 103, 105
Polanski, Roman. 64–5, 68

Rank, O. 102
Reed, Carol. 60
Reid, K. 154, 158
Reik, T. 102
Rogers, Carl. 108, 115, 130
Rorty, R. 63, 68
Roth, W.D. 180, 182, 191
Rosenhan, D. 104, 109
Rush, Benjamin. 72, 81
Rushdie, S. 148, 159

Sartre, J-P. 11
Sachs, H. 103
Seligman, M. 103
Shapiro, M. 104
Shaw, G.B. 5
St William of Norwich 61
Staub, E. 104, 109
Sutherland, J. 59, 66, 68
Szasz, T. S. 78, 84

Terman, L.M. 5, 15

Waititi, Taika. 116–7, 128
Wechsler, D. 104, 108
Weinberg, G. 104
West, W. 133, 141, 144, 145
Wolpe, J. 104

Zola, Emile. 106

Subject index

Aboriginal and Torres Strait Islander 12, 14, 44, 55–6
Acta Psychologica Sinica 8
Adinkra symbols 4, 13, 35, 38
African Americans 5, 9–10, 38, 76, 77, 176
American Medico-Psychological Association 72
American Psychiatric Association 7, 72, 73
American Psychological Association 8, 9, 72, 75, 83
Ananse stories 4, 35, 37
Annual Conference Against Psychiatric Oppression and on Human Rights 71, 81
Anosognosia 70
anti-Semitism 16–7, 22, 24, 25, 57, 58, 61, 64, 67, 99, 106, 107
Aotearoa 110–130
appearance 22–3
Ashkenazim 22, 25, 65, 66, 69
Assertive Community Treatment 75–6, 83
Assisted Outpatient Treatment 78, 83
Association of
  Black Psychologists (ABPsi) 9–10, 36
  Medical Superintendents of American Insane Institutions 72, 82
assumptions 32, 51, 53, 126, 135
  cultural 43, 141, 150, 154
Auschwitz 64, 103
Australia 3, 43–56
Australian
  Indigenous Psychology Education Project (AIPEP) 48–9, 51, 53
  Psychological Society 55
    Apology 12, 14, 47, 55
Autoethnography 133–134, 142, 143
Ayurvedic medicine 4

belt
  and braces 34
Big Brother 27, 37
binary
  opposition 153
  thinking 132–133, 142
biochemical imbalance 4
biomedical model 131–132, 133, 141
Bipolar disorder 21, 25 (*see also* nonsense)
Black
  African and Asian Therapy Network (BAATN) 11–4, 131
  And Minority Ethnic (BAME) 9, 11, 13, 15, 86, 90–6, 131–133, 142, 191
  Lives Matter 28, 34, 39, 96
Blood libel 57, 61
brainwashing 112
Brexit 25, 26, 41, 134, 139–140, 143, 147, 188
British Association for Counselling and Psychotherapy (BACP) 131, 132, 142, 167

Calcutta 6, 149, 151
censorship 67
Chinese Psychological Society 8, 13
circumcision 134, 138–139, 143
class 4, 6, 10, 26, 31, 38, 39, 52, 102, 143, 149, 161, 166, 181, 185, 190
Clinical Psychology Forum 12, 14
Close the Gap (CtG) 45
colonialism 27, 37, 42, 100, 132
colonisation 42, 44–6, 53, 111, 112, 116, 118, 143
  de- 119, 120, 143
  psychology as 117
colour
  blindness 178, 186, 187, 190

people of 11, 71, 78–9, 81, 82, 87, 136, 148, 149, 156, 160, 165, 177, 188
community 3, 12, 20, 21, 63, 66, 77, 94, 97, 121, 123, 127, 184, 190
connectedness 34
compliance 44, 70, 94
context 12, 29, 81, 133, 150, 151, 180, 183, 184
Critical
Appraisal Skills Programme (CASP) 181, 189
Race Theory 30, 34, 126
cultural
bias 30, 34, 126
sensitivity 91, 148, 152, 158
culture
mixed 133
transculturalism 98, 130

decolonizing
curriculum 43–4, 119–122
profession 122–123
practitioner 123–127
diagnosis 88
Diagnostic and Statistical Manual (DSM) 7, 74
difference 92, 161
disability 31, 71, 88–9, 90, 92, 94, 164
diversity 6, 9–10, 15, 87, 92, 113, 161
politics 166
strategy 33
Division of Clinical Psychology 10, 92, 100
Special Interest Group in Race and Culture 9–10
symposium 87, 109
Down's Syndrome 5, 88
drapetomania 73, 74, 81
dysesthesia 73

East India Company 6, 73
education
project 47
selective 89
epistemology 111, 118–119, 123, 126
exclusion 87, 106, 166
expectations 70, 122, 136, 137, 157

First Nations 45
Fugitive Slave Act (1793) 81

Gabai 104
gender 31, 70, 76, 94, 138, 159, 165, 166, 169, 183
reassignment 164
genocide 5, 44, 104, 109
Genthanasia 5
Gnatentod 107

healing 4, 6, 11, 27, 35
Health Practitioners Competence Assurance Amendment Act 2020 115
hell 10, 11
heteronormative 163, 167–8
Hinduism 11 29, 37
HOMMS 29, 37
hospitality 115
hospitalization 76–7

identity 45, 46, 74, 95, 112–113, 125, 133, 135, 142, 149, 160–173, 180, 182–186
Ifaluk 3
India Education (website) 6–7, 14
Indian Association of Clinical Psychology 7
Indian Psychological Association 6
Indian Journal of Clinical Psychology 7, 15
Indigenising the Curriculum (ItC) 43–4, 51, 53–4
Indigenous 3, 43–54, 109, 111, 119
psychology 47, 94, 112, 123
individualism 5, 11, 12, 94, 132, 150
Institute for Jewish Policy Research 18
intersectionality 88, 165, 180, 185
invisibility 23–4, 133
Israel 16, 17, 19, 23–4

Jewish
American Princess (JAP) 22
Theological Seminary of America 58
Jewishness 22–4, 65
Journal
of Curriculum Studies 120
of Insanity 80
Judaism 4, 11, 100, 102, 106
and criminality 106, 107
jüdischer Gauner 106

Kemetic 27, 37
Kōhanga Reo 111, 112
Kura Kaupapa Māori 111, 112

language 8–9, 91, 92, 115, 111, 117, 134–135, 149
racist 187
Learning Disability Partnership Board 96
liminality 139, 144
Lunatics Liberation Movement 70

Maafa 26, 27, 37
Māori
  immersion pre-school 111–112
  names 116
medical model 131–132
Medieval mystery plays 59
Mental Patients Liberation Movement 69
microaggression 33, 41
migration 34, 95, 113, 139, 143, 147, 155
murder 27, 33, 57, 60, 61–2, 69, 102, 103, 106
music 64, 135, 168

name 102, 116, 134, 136, 137–138, 143, 144, 163, 180
Nationalism 28, 33, 147, 169
Native Schools Act 111
Nazi 18, 23, 66, 103
Neoliberalism 132, 146
New wave 133, 142
Ngā Tama Toa 111
Nguzo Saba 35
non-expert position 158
nonsense (see bipolar disorder and Obsessive Compulsive Disorder)

objectification 132, 171, 173
Opo, the friendly dolphin 110
Obsessive Compulsive Disorder (OCD) – *see also* nonsense 20, 24
Oedipus complex 104
oppression 29, 31, 33, 69–76, 81–2, 87, 161, 165, 177, 183, 184, 186–187
  psychiatric 69–71, 76
Otherness 164, 165, 172
  the other 12, 34, 115, 162–173

Pākehā 110–112
Paris 162
Pasifika 113–114, 117
  diaspora 113
paternalism 44–5, 51
perceptions 30, 136, 138
Pintupi 3
post racial 178, 186–187, 190
protectionism 44–5, 49
psychiatric
  survivor movement 69–71
Psychology
  African 4, 26–7, 34
    centred 35
  Afrikan 35
  Clinical 7, 10, 12, 26–36, 86–94, 112, 147, 176–188
  Educational 35
  History of 3, 22, 50, 117
Psychotherapy 10, 22, 105, 108, 115, 146, 152, 158, 172
  Counselling and 12, 132, 142, 160, 167
  Family 152, 154
  Improving Access to Psychological Therapies (IAPT) programme 132, 148
  Systemic 152
  Therapeutic relationship 125, 131, 158

Qualitative research 32, 152, 153

Rabbi/*rebbe* 4, 104, 108
racial inconsistency 179–181, 185–188
racism
  Institutional 4, 27–8, 33–4, 91
reconciliation 48–54
reparation 26, 74
resilience 28, 31, 47, 127, 156
rituals 21, 35, 61, 89, 106, 115, 139, 152
  rites of passage 136

Saltpêtrière 106
self-knowledge 36, 70
Sephardim 66
sexism 88, 173
shoplifting 177
Slavery 66, 69, 72, 74, 78, 80, 176
  psychiatric 78, 79, 81
Social
  Darwinism 43, 46, 106
  media 18, 28
solutions 43
spirit and spirituality 4, 6, 33, 35, 37, 70, 81, 94, 111, 121, 124, 165
spiritus nullius 54
stereotyping 90, 93, 94, 137
supervision 27, 35, 126
suicide 8, 101, 118

Tāngata whenua 110, 118
television 57, 64
Te reo 111, 114, 115
Terman-Merrill Index 5
Thirteenth Amendment 79, 80
Tohunga Suppression Act 1907 18, 130
trauma 28, 46, 111, 139
Treaty of Waitangi 112, 114, 119, 120, 124, 126, 130
Tsitzis 24
Turkish 133–141
  nose 136

Ubuntu 34, 40
University 19–20, 23, 27, 52–3, 113, 119
Utica
  Crib 70
  State Lunatic Asylum 70, 80

vibration 27, 34, 35

welfarism 44
Whānaungatanga 124–125
whipping – as cure 72–3
  see also drapetomania
White
  fragility 32, 170
  supremacy 26, 28, 31, 34, 36, 74, 168, 170, 176, 188
  whiteness 29, 31, 32, 74, 96, 167, 176, 179
Windrush 27, 39, 171
Winterbourne scandal 95, 96
Woke 27, 37
workplace 28, 29, 32, 168

yarmulke 23
Yom Kippur 23, 100
Youth Rights Movement 69